CONTENTS

INTRODUCTION

Are you ready for the fragrance of the juicy bit of red meat as it starts to frizzle on your grill?

Are you ready to feel the softness of the same piece and the release of the tasty juiciness?

I've always been, it is my passion, my hobby and, now more than ever, also my job.

It doesn't matter what is your favorite food. If it is not liquid, almost certainly, cooked on a grill, it will taste better. (And if it cannot be cooked on a grill, it's time you get yourself a versatile griddle. By chance I've got the best guide to help you with that, here:).

Whether you're preparing chicken breasts, steaks, or a variety of garden-fresh vegetables and fruits, you can make your friends' taste buds go over the moon, if you know what you're doing.

Grilling is a unique cooking process that often involves grilling meals outdoor over a preheated grill. It has evolved in various ways over time and has also become a favorite summer cooking method. What's even better, grilled dishes are often nutritious and healthier than those cooked on the stove with oil. Grilling food is a great way to reduce weight because the fat on meat melts and drips off the grill, lowering your chances of consuming dangerous saturated fats.

We all know grilling is a fun activity that you can do with your friends and family in your backyard. It's a relaxing way to eat in an open-air atmosphere where children may play sports & adults can interact while enjoying wonderful food and drinks. To put it another way, grilling is fun, and where the grill & food combo is involved everybody has a great time. Grilling is the best way to introduce fresh dishes during the summer, so take advantage of it while you can.

This cookbook contains delicious dishes that will inspire anyone to become a Pitmaster. You will find all of the classic hibachi recipes, such as fried rice and stirs fry, as well as a range of unexpectedly great ideas. Remember that these are unique recipes, so be open to trying new things. Also, keep in mind that the cooking method in this cookbook is simple. So, while the meals will be distinctive and delicious, they will be simple to prepare.

CHAPTER 1: LET'S GRILL

Cooking outside is a global pleasure. During festivities and events that involve outdoor grills and barbeques, many great memories are made. The aroma of grilled meat in the air, mixed with the sensation of being encircled by friends and family, makes for a memorable event.

Nothing beats a good whole-hearted BBQ in summer time, and choosing "grilled" dishes over "fried" meals is one of the golden laws of eating healthily: because there's no batter dripping or coating oil on grilled food, it's a healthier option.

1.1 WHAT IS A GRILL?

Cooking food on a grill entails introducing it to direct heat. Both gas and electricity can be used as heat sources. However, there are some differences between the griddle and the grill.

Most of us are familiar with what a grill is but for those newbies out there who are not familiar with barbequeing, here are some of the significant points you should know about grills.

1. Cooking Surface

A grill is made of cast iron grates or stainless steel or open spaces between them to let the oils and fats from the meal drain away in their most basic form. A bigger flat plate with elevated ridges is used in modern closed design grills.

2. Typical Uses

Grills are the preferred solution for steaks, sandwiches, hamburgers, chops, and most vegetables. If you wish to give your food a lovely smoky flavor and some great grill marks, grills are ideal. However, you won't be able to cook items that start as liquids, such as pancakes, if you use typical grills with open wires. If you wish to cook that kind of food use a griddle instead.

3. Cooking Temperature

Be aware that a typical grill cooks at temperatures in the range of 400 ° F, which is substantially higher than the 350 ° F that a griddle cooks at.

The food will use greater temperatures if you use a typical open-style grill. This reduces the possibility of flare-ups and thus makes them safer to use.

4. Ideal Place to Use It

In addition to producing a lot of heat, grills also emit a lot of smoke when cooking, making them ideal for outdoor cooking. On the other hand, many modern grills are designed primarily for indoor usage and have a more effective ventilation system.

5. Food Texture and Taste

Grilled dishes will have a somewhat burnt flavor and a charred texture, as well as some appealing grill marks. When using coal or charcoal pellet-powered grills, this texture and flavor will be even more noticeable.

6. Buying and Ownership Cost

Grills are usually quite cheap, but the price will vary depending on the style, size, and fuel source. The less expensive are generally the charcoal versions, which will have the lowest ownership costs.

CHAPTER 2: THE GRILL

Grills are real cooking classics and one of the greatest and most freely accessible forms of outdoor cookers. Over a heating surface, they commonly have cast iron or stainless steel grates. The signature pattern sear marks on burger steaks are formed by these grates, which is one of the many reasons why people prefer grills.

Grills generate heat from beneath the food; however, this varies depending on the style of the grill. Almost all grills are designed to use one of three fuel sources: gas, charcoal, gas, or wood pellets. The principle is the same regardless of the fuel source. To create a hot, uniform, constant cooking environment for your food, start a flame or fire below the meal and close the lid.

3.1 DIFFERENT TYPES OF GRILLS

1. Gas Grills

It is the most common form of the grill for use in the backyard. They can be powered by either bottled natural gas or propane from your local utility. Although most gas grills are intended for propane, they can readily be changed to natural gas. Some people debate whether propane or methane is better, although there isn't much of a difference. If you have accessibility to a natural gas connection, using it instead of propane tanks is surely handier and less expensive.

Advantages: The hurried chef wants to fire up the grill and prepare dinner without dealing with charcoal setup and cleanup.

Disadvantages: Both in terms of taste and price. Although some gas grills include small smoker boxes, you'll only receive a tiny little bit of the smoke taste you'd get from a real charcoal smoker or grill. While some low-cost gas grills, the processes guarantee that they will always cost more than just a comparable charcoal grill.

2. Charcoal Grills

These grills cook with charcoal briquettes as fuel and a source of heat. Cooking with charcoal takes longer and costs more than cooking with gas, but some users will always like the smell of charcoal, especially if it is made of natural wood.

Advantages: A charcoal grill is the only way to obtain both a Smokey grilled flavor and the pleasure of smoking meats. Because charcoal burns at such a higher temperature than gas, an experienced grill master can sear the meat quickly. Finally, cooking with charcoal has a certain romance to it that a modern gas grill lacks.

Disadvantages; The amount of time and money required, as well as the cost of charcoal. You can't just light a charcoal barbecue and throw something on it. Beginning the coals & pre-heating the grill takes at least 40 mins to get it ready to use. When you're finished cooking, you'll need to clean up the grill and dispose of the ashes. When compared to gas, buying charcoal is also fairly costly.

3. Electric Grills

These grills are electrically powered and use hot grill plates for cooking meat. There are both indoor and outdoor options.

Advantages: People in the cities who cannot use charcoal or gas grills due to fire laws. Check out your local laws & building codes to ensure that the grill you purchase complies with them.

Disadvantages: Electric grills can generate results that resemble those of their gas-powered counterparts (grill marks are common), but they are not a substitute for a regular grill. When using electricity, the Smokey flavor is almost completely lost.

4. Smoker grill

A smoker grill is built to smoke meat in a horizontal, long chamber that rests beside the heat source instead of directly above it, making it much easier to regulate the heat and replace the fuel because you don't have to move food out of the way to add wood or coals to the heat source.

Meat can be smoked in two ways. Cold smoking is the first method, which works best with chicken breast, pork chops, beef, sausage, salmon, steak, scallops, and cheese. Cold smoking occurs when the temperature is between 68 - 86 ° F. Cold smoking is mostly utilized for flavor, and it's normally done on meat that's already been cured or cooked.

When you want to properly cook the food you're smoking while also imparting that great smoky taste, hot smoking is the way to go. The temperature range for hot smoking is 126°F – 176°F. Meat shrinkage and buckling can occur when hot smoking is done at temperatures above 185°F. Large chunks of meat, such as ham, ribs, ham hocks, pulled pork, and brisket, benefit from hot smoking. Hot smoked meats are usually reheated or cooked additional later, but they are safe to eat right away if thoroughly cooked through. Hot smoking imparts moisture to the meat and aids in the preservation of its natural tastes.

5. Pellet grills

Pellet grills have quickly become the biggest trend in the grilling and BBQ world. People are pleased about the additional conveniences and features that pellet grills offer to the market, especially since innovation in the industry hasn't progressed much over the last thirty years or so. However, understanding how they work is essential to fully enjoy everything they have to offer.

Pellet grills are outdoor burners that combine smokers, charcoal and gas grills, and ovens into one unit. How do pellet grills work?

Wood pellets are placed into a hopper, which serves as a storage container. A pellet smoker involves heating a cooking chamber in which air circulates, convectively heating food. Food is cooked on grill grates toward the top of the cooking chamber, while hardwood or charcoal pellets burn at the bottom. More wood is delivered from a pellet hopper situated above the cooking chamber when the fuel supply runs low. These pellets are pushed down a chute and into the chamber's heart by an auger.

Airflow controls the temperature settings on such a pellet smoker. Heavy-duty fans towards the bottom of the unit draw air into the lower section of the cooking chamber, where oxygen is absorbed by the burning pellets, increasing the temperature. Meanwhile, when the top cover of the smoker is opened, the heat might escape.

How to use a pellet grill?

Prepare your pellet smoker by seasoning it

We must first season the smoker before continuing. This is an important step for any new smoker since it protects them from the harmful effects of long-term continuous use. The basic notion is to coat the grates and the inside of the chamber in cooking oil, then run the smoker without food for a 'dry run.' This will cook the oil into the smoker's interior surfaces, providing a protective layer.

After you've finished seasoning it, let it cool and settle for at least one day before using it.

Preheat your smoker

The problem with charcoal grills is that they take a long time to heat up. It can be not easy to light them and keep them at a comfortable temperature. With a pellet grill, this is not the case. They operate similarly to an oven.

Switch on your grill by plugging it into an electrical outlet or socket and setting your desired temperature. If you want to smoke meat on the grill, set the temperature to 225°F.

To warm and get to temperature, most smokers will take about ten minutes. As the smoker heats up, you should hear a low rumble from it. This is your smoker's motorized auger or firebox coming to life, and it's a good sign that it's working & warming up.

While pellet smokers include a temperature gauge on its control display, it's not uncommon for it to be off by up to 20°F in either direction. Get a thermometer with two probes for your smoker. These help to monitor both cooking and interior meat temperatures at the same time. The most accurate models outperform the bulk of built-in gauges.

Add your meat

Put the meat on the smoker grates carefully once your pellet smoker has reached the desired temperature. Place the meal in the center of the grate for the best results. This keeps the meat far enough away from the heat to avoid drying out yet close enough to cook at the proper temperature.

Keep an eye on the fat content

The meat itself is a common blunder made by many newbies to BBQ. Meat that is too thin can dry out rapidly, but meat with too much fat can obstruct the smoke's ability to penetrate the meat's body.

If you're going to smoke any cut like brisket, make sure the fat layer is about 12 inches thick before placing it on the smoker.

3.2 SEASON YOUR GRILL

Your grill is contaminated with oils and chemicals from the factory where it was built, which emit foul smoke and ruin the quality of any food you cook. It's all about burning it off before it goes on your meal when you season it.

Seasoning a grill is a basic procedure that involves oiling and preheating your grill before using it for the first time. There are numerous advantages to this, including the removal of hazardous manufacturing pollutants.

Seasoning is beneficial for all new grills, whether charcoal or gas, cast iron or stainless steel. Take these easy steps.

- Rinse, and air dry the grill grates completely. Dish soap isn't required. If you do, make sure to rinse and dry them completely.
- Clean the grates all over with a high heat resistant oil such as vegetable oil, peanut oil, or canola oil, using a basting brush or maybe even a clean paintbrush or paper towel. It's also good to use a spray bottle of oil or maybe even a can of Pam.
- Brush or wipe the oil inside the lid, the insides of the pit, and, if your grill has them, the emitters. The idea is to bake the grates and grill and seal them. The oil will enter into the cast iron pores, bake in, harden, and form a smooth non-stick covering that will darken and enhance with each use.
- Light your charcoal or turn up the heat on your gas. It would help if you had your grill to be scorching.
- Allow 30-40 minutes for it to burn, smoke, and work its high-heat magic.

3.3 SEASONING'S ADVANTAGES

1. Easier Cooking and cleaning

Seasoning will make non-stick cooking easier and allow your grill to perform at its best. This is because cooking oils and fats attach to the grates and produce a smooth non-stick surface over time. This is especially important for cast iron grates, which are porous and absorb oils and fats. Non-stick surfaces, of course, make cleanup a pleasure.

Better Flavor

When you grill, the fluids and fats from the food evaporate and cover the whole inside surface of your grill, including the grates, lid, pit, and everything else, giving it that unique grill flavor. Every time you light it up, the flavor becomes better and better.

2. Lasts longer

Finally, treating your grill will extend its life and keep it from rusting.

If you season your grill regularly, you'll get years of superb grilling and taste out of it.

3.4 MAINTENANCE

- Before turning on the grill, lightly coat the grate with just a high-smoking temperature oil like peanut oil to prevent food from sticking. The cooking spray also helps.
- When grills are slightly warm, they clean up best. After cooking, use a ball of aluminum foil or a wire brush held between tongs to scrape the grate. On stainless steel grates, use brass wire brushes; on cast iron, use stainless steel wire brushes.
- Clean up spills with a damp paper towel after the grill has cooled completely. Corrosion is accelerated by oil and salt.
- After the ashes have cooled, throw them out on a charcoal grill. Clean or replace the catch-pan liner on gas grills regularly.
- After each usage, cover your grill with a water-resistant cover.

3.5 ESSENTIAL TIPS

1. Begin with a squeaky-clean grill: Don't let the salmon skin from yesterday night's dinner give a fishy-char taste to tonight's chicken breasts. In between uses, clean the grates with a robust metal brush. It's simplest to do this when the grill is hot.)

2. Do not mix the food: The fewer times you flip anything, the better in general. Allow the meat to cook a little longer if it's stuck to the grill; it'll unstick itself when it's time to flip it.

3. Have a spray bottle on hand in case of a flare-up: Flames aren't your food's buddies; they'll scorch it in an unappealing way. Keep a spray bottle full of water available to cool down flare-ups without messing with the heat.

4. Buy a meat thermometer: It isn't easy to detect meat temperature simply by touching it unless you're a very skilled cook. (However, if you're curious, here's how to accomplish it: Maintain contact with the meat. It's unusual if it's soft, like the flesh between your index and thumb. It's medium-rare if it's soft, like your cheek, and well-done if it's firm, like your forehead.)

5. Don't place cold meals directly on the grill: Allowing the meat to come to room temperature on the table for thirty min before grilling aids in even cooking. (However, if you want a rare sear for example, if you're grilling tuna, then chilled is the way to go)

6. Slightly undercook your meals: Carryover cooking occurs when food continues to cook after it has been removed from the grill. After leaving the grill, the temperature of the food will rise by around five degrees, so prepare appropriately.

7. Allow all meat to rest: Allow the meat to rest for 10-15 minutes after cooking, undisturbed (and unsliced!). This will enable the juices to redistribute. The longer the rest time, the larger the chunk of meat. Resting meat is essential for juicy outcomes.

8. If you want to cook meat thoroughly with bones, don't over-char it: No one wants to eat meat with a thick layer of black char on it. Cook thicker bone-in meats, such as chicken legs, on high heat for a nice crust before moving to a lower, indirect fire on the grill. This will enable the meat to cook through much more slowly while preventing the outside from becoming overcooked. Alternatively, pre-cook the chicken for 20 to 30 minutes in the oven before grilling. Ribs are also nice to prepare ahead of time. When serving a large group, keep things simple. Managing multiple cook times for various proteins and vegetables can quickly become difficult, resulting in mistakes and overcooking. Reduce the number of protein alternatives as much as feasible, and provide variety in the form of unusual side dishes, sauces, or condiments.

CHAPTER 3: GRILL RECIPES

PART 1: PORK RECIPES

Grilled Pork Tenderloins

(Ready in about 30 minutes | serving 4|Difficulty: Easy)

Per serving: Kcal 196, Fat: 4g, Net Carbs: 15g, Protein: 24g

Ingredients

- Honey 1/3 cup
- Soy sauce 1/3 cup, reduced-sodium
- Teriyaki sauce 1/3 cup
- Brown sugar 3 tbsp.
- Gingerroot 1 tbsp., fresh & minced
- Garlic 3 cloves, minced
- Ketchup 4 tsp
- Onion powder ½ tsp
- Cinnamon ½ tsp, ground
- Cayenne pepper ¼ tsp
- 1 lb. pork tenderloins 2
- Cooked rice

Instructions

1. Mix the first ten ingredients in a large mixing bowl. Half of the marinade should be poured into a bowl, and then the tenderloins should be tossed to coat. Cover and chill for 6-8 hours or overnight, flipping the pork as needed. Cover and keep the remaining marinade refrigerated.

2. Drain the pork and discard out the marinade. Grill for 20-35 minutes, covered, over indirect medium-high heat, until a thermometer reaches 145° F, occasionally turning and basting with remaining marinade. Allow for 5 minutes of resting time before slicing. Serve with a bowl of rice.

Smoked Pork Butt

(Ready in about 22 hours| serving 4|Difficulty: Difficult)
Per serving: Kcal 321, Fat: 21.6g, Net Carbs: 3.3g, Protein: 26.5g

Ingredients
- 7 lbs. Pork butt roast, fresh
- Ground Chile powder 2 tbsp.
- 4 tbsp. Brown sugar, packed

Instructions
1. Soak the pork butt for at least 3 hours or overnight in a brine solution if desired. Preheat the grill to 200 - 225 degrees F.
2. Mix the chili powder, brown sugar, and any other seasonings to taste in a small bowl. Add generously to meat, then rub it with your fingers. Place the pork on a roasting rack that has been placed in a drip pan.
3. Grill for 6 - 12 hours at 200 - 225 degrees F, or till inner pork temperature reaches 145 degrees F.

World's Best Honey Garlic Pork Chops

(Ready in about 25 minutes | serving 4|Difficulty: Easy)
Per serving: Kcal 208, Fat: 5.6g, Net Carbs: 13.5g, Protein: 25.6g

Ingredients
- Ketchup ½ cup
- Honey 2 ⅔ tbsp.
- 2 tbsp. soy sauce, low-sodium
- Garlic 2 cloves, crushed
- 6 pork chops, 4 ounces

Instructions
1. Preheat the grill to medium heat and brush the grate gently with oil.
2. To prepare a glaze, combine ketchup, soy sauce, honey, and garlic in a bowl.
3. On a hot grill, sear the pork chops on both sides. Brush a thin layer of glaze on each side of chops as they cook, and grill until the center is no longer pink, about 7–9 minutes per side. The temperature should read 145 degrees F on an instant-read thermometer placed into the center.

Fiery Pork Skewers

(Ready in about 30 minutes | serving 4|Difficulty: Easy)

Per serving: Kcal 147, Fat: 4.8g, Net Carbs: 3g, Protein: 18.1g

Ingredients

- Teriyaki sauce 2 tbsp.
- Red wine vinegar 1 tbsp.
- Vegetable oil 1 tbsp.
- Brown sugar 1 tsp
- Flakes of red pepper ½ tsp
- Pork tenderloin ¾ lbs., sliced into 1-inch cubes

Instructions

1. Combine teriyaki sauce, vegetable oil, red wine vinegar, brown sugar, and red pepper flakes in a medium mixing bowl. Cubes of pork tenderloin should be added to the mixture. Toss to evenly coat.

2. Preheat an outside grill to high heat and brush the grate gently with oil.

3. Put the pork on skewers. Cook on a preheated grill, rotating frequently and coating with the teriyaki sauce mixture. Cook for 12 - 15 minutes, or until the desired doneness is achieved.

Ham and Pineapple Kabobs

(Ready in about 25 minutes | serving 4|Difficulty: Easy)

Per serving: Kcal 342, Fat: 19.3g, Net Carbs: 26.8g, Protein: 16.2g

Ingredients

- Brown sugar 3 tbsp.
- White vinegar 2 tbsp., distilled
- Vegetable oil 1 tbsp.
- Prepared mustard 1 tsp
- Cooked ham ¾ lbs. , sliced into 1-inch cubes
- 1 can drain pineapple chunks, 15 ounces
- Skewers

Instructions

1. Preheat the grill to high.

2. Combine brown sugar, vegetable oil, vinegar, and mustard in a medium mixing bowl.
 Using skewers, alternately thread pineapple and ham slices.

3. Oil the grill grate lightly. Brush the skewers well with brown sugar mix before placing them on the heated grill. Cook for 6 - 8 minutes, flipping and basting regularly. When thoroughly cooked and thickly glazed, serve it.

Chili Crusted Pork Tenderloin

(Ready in about 35 minutes | serving 4|Difficulty: Easy)

Per serving: Kcal 183, Fat: 6.1g, Net Carbs: 11.7g, Protein: 20.4g

Ingredients

- Onion powder 1 tsp
- Garlic powder 1 tsp
- Chipotle Chile powder 3 tbsp.
- Salt 1 ½ tsp
- Brown sugar 4 tbsp.
- 2 pork tenderloins ¾ lbs.

Instructions

1. Preheat the grill to medium-high.
2. Mix the onion powder, salt, chipotle Chile powder, garlic powder, and brown sugar in a big resealable plastic bag. Place the tenderloins in the bag and shake to evenly coat the pork. Put it in the fridge for 15 minutes.
3. Lightly oil the grill grate and place the pork on it. Cook the pork for 20 minutes, flipping every 5 minutes. Remove it from the grill and set aside for 5 - 10 minutes before slicing.

Tropical Grilled Pork Chops

(Ready in about 2 hours | serving 4|Difficulty: Moderate)

Per serving: Kcal 269, Fat: 7.2g, Net Carbs: 37.1g, Protein: 15.1g

Ingredients

- Garlic 1 clove, minced
- Chili powder 1 tsp
- Cayenne pepper ¼ tsp
- Cardamom seeds, 1 pod
- Water ½ tsp, or as needed
- Vegetable oil 1 tsp
- Rice wine vinegar ¼ cup
- Sugar ½ cup
- Mango 1, peeled & chopped
- Salt ¼ tsp
- Cilantro ½ tsp
- Lemon juice 2 tsp
- Jalapeno pepper 1, minced & fresh
- Applesauce 1 ½ cups, unsweetened
- Pineapple 3 rings, chopped
- White pepper 1 pinch
- Soy sauce ⅓ cup
- Rice wine vinegar ⅓ cup
- Pork chops 6

Instructions

2.   Mash the garlic, cayenne, chili powder, and cardamom seeds together in a mortar and pestle. Pour in just enough water to make a paste.

3.   In a saucepan, heat the oil over medium heat. Cook, constantly stirring, until the spice paste starts to bubble, around 30 seconds. Cook for 2 minutes without boiling after adding the vinegar. Stir in the sugar until it is completely dissolved. Simmer for 20 minutes after adding the mango, cilantro, salt, lemon juice, and jalapeno. Cook for another 10 minutes after adding the applesauce and pineapple. Add White pepper for taste. Refrigerate till ready to use in a bowl with a cover.

4.   To make the marinade, combine 1/3 cup soy sauce, 2/3 cup salsa, and 1/3 cup vinegar. Pour the marinade over the pork chops in a big resealable plastic bag. Refrigerate for 1 hour after tightly sealing the bag.

5.   Preheat the grill to medium-high. Drain the marinade from the bag and bring it to a boil in a saucepan.

6.   Oil the grill grate lightly. Preheat the grill and place the pork chops on it. Cook for 10 minutes, or until the desired doneness is reached, flipping once and basting with the boiling marinade as needed.

7.   Over medium-low heat, reheat the remaining salsa. Serve the pork chops with the salsa on top.

Martha's Magic Meat Rub Pork Roast

(Ready in about 4 hours 30 minutes | serving 4|Difficulty: Difficult)

Per serving: Kcal 282, Fat: 16.8g, Net Carbs: 3.2g, Protein: 28.4g

Ingredients

- Adobo seasoning 2 tbsp.
- Red pepper flakes ½ tbsp., crushed
- Chili powder 2 tsp
- Celery salt 2 tsp
- Black pepper 1 tsp, ground
- 1 pork shoulder roast, 4 lbs., boneless & butterflied
- Bacon 6 slices
- Onions 9 green

Instructions

1. Make sure the grill is set up for indirect heat.
2. Combine crushed red pepper, adobo seasoning, celery salt, chili powder, and black pepper in a mixing bowl. Rub the mixture all over the roast.
3. Place the bacon strips (uncooked) on a flat surface and topped with 3 green onions. Put the roast on top of the green onions and bacon. On top of the roast, place 3 green onions. Fold the roast over carefully, wrapping it with bacon strips & green onions, and securing it with kitchen twine.
4. Inside the grill, set up a drip pan and lightly oil the grill grate. Place the roast over the drip pan on the grill grate and top with the remaining green onions. Cover and cook for 4 hours over indirect heat to a minimum internal temperature of 145 degrees F.

Simple Country Ribs

(Ready in about 1 hour 10 minutes | serving 4|Difficulty: Easy)

Per serving: Kcal 882, Fat: 38.3g, Net Carbs: 94.1g, Protein: 36.4g

Ingredients

- Pork spareribs 2 ½ lbs.
- 2 bottles barbeque sauce 18 ounces
- Onion 1, quartered
- Salt 1 tsp
- Black pepper ½ tsp, ground

Instructions

1. In a large stockpot, combine spareribs, onion, barbecue sauce, pepper and salt. Fill with just enough water to cover it. Bring to a low boil, then reduce to low heat and simmer for about 40 minutes.
2. Preheat the grill to high.
3. Grates should be lightly oiled. Place the spareribs on the grill after removing them from the stockpot. During the cooking process, baste the ribs with the barbeque sauce in the saucepan. Grill the ribs for 20 minutes, basting and regularly flipping, until it's nicely browned.

Glenn's Marinated Pork Shoulder

(Ready in about 7 hours 15 minutes | serving 6|Difficulty: Difficult)

Per serving: Kcal 497, Fat: 21.4g, Net Carbs: 12.9g, Protein: 58.6g

Ingredients

- Garlic ¼ cup, chopped
- Onion ½ cup, chopped
- Soy sauce 1 dash
- Corn syrup 1 tbsp.
- Apple juice 2 tbsp.
- Worcestershire sauce 3 tbsp.
- Molasses 1 tsp
- Wine ¼ cup
- Salad dressing ¼ cup, Italian-style
- White vinegar ½ cup, distilled
- Garlic powder ½ tsp
- Salt 1/8 tsp
- Onion powder ½ tsp
- Cajun seasoning 1 tbsp.
- Red pepper ½ tsp crushed
- Seasoning salt ¼ tsp
- Brown sugar ¼ cup
- Pork shoulder 8 lbs.

Instructions

1. Mix garlic, soy sauce, onion, corn syrup, apple juice, molasses, Worcestershire sauce, wine, distilled white vinegar, Italian-style salad dressing, garlic powder, salt, Cajun spice, onion powder, crushed red pepper, seasoned salt, and brown sugar together in a large mixing bowl.

2. Pork shoulder should be sliced 1/8 – 1/4 inch deep. Add to the marinade mixture in the mixing bowl. Refrigerate the marinade for at least 4 hours.

3. Preheat an outdoor grill to medium-high and lightly oil the grill grate.

4. Cook the marinated pork shoulder for 3 hours on a preheated grill or until it reaches a minimum internal temperature of 165 degrees F. While grilling, brush with the marinade frequently.

Char Siu (Chinese BBQ Pork)

(Ready in about 3 hours 40 minutes | serving 4|Difficulty: Difficult)

Per serving: Kcal 483, Fat: 8.9g, Net Carbs: 53.5g, Protein: 43.8g

Ingredients

- Pork tenderloins 2
- Soy sauce ½ cup
- Honey ⅓ cup
- Ketchup ⅓ cup
- Brown sugar ⅓ cup
- Chinese rice wine ¼ cup
- Hoisin sauce 2 tbsp.
- Food color, red ½ tsp (optional)
- Chinese spice powder 1 tsp (optional)

Instructions

1. Cut the pork into 1 1/2- to 2-inch-long strips with grain and place them in a big resealable plastic bag.

2. In a saucepan over medium heat, combine soy sauce, rice wine, honey, brown sugar, red food coloring, ketchup, hoisin sauce, and Chinese five-spice powder. Cook, constantly stirring, for 2 to 3 minutes, or mixed and slightly heated. Fill the bag with pork and the marinade, squeeze out the air, and seal it. Turn the bag a few times to ensure that all pork chunks are covered in the marinade.

3. Refrigerate the pork for 2 hours overnight.

4. Preheat the outdoor grill to medium-high heat and brush the grate liberally with oil.

5. Remove the pork from the marinade and shake it to get rid of any extra liquid. Remove and discard any remaining marinade.

6. Cook the pork for 20 minutes on a hot grill. Place a small container of water on the grill and continue to cook, flipping the pork frequently, for about 1 hour, or until it is cooked through. At least 145 degrees F should be read on an instant-read thermometer placed into the center.

Marinated Pork Tenderloin with Garlic- Maple

(Ready in about 8 hours 30 minutes | serving 4|Difficulty: Difficult)

Per serving: Kcal 288, Fat: 4.9g, Net Carbs: 36.8g, Protein: 23.5g

Ingredients

- Dijon mustard 2 tbsp.
- Sesame oil 1 tsp
- Maple syrup, 1 cup
- Black pepper, freshly ground, to taste
- Pork tenderloin 1 ½ lb.
- Garlic 3 cloves, minced

Instructions

1. Mix the sesame oil, mustard, pepper, garlic, & maple syrup in a mixing bowl. Place the pork in a small bowl and marinate it completely. Cover and chill for at least 8 hours or overnight in the refrigerator.
2. Preheat the grill to medium-low.
3. Set aside the pork after removing it from the marinade. Transfer the leftover marinade to a small saucepan and simmer for 5 minutes on the stove over medium heat.
4. Brush the grate with oil before placing the pork on it. Grill pork for 15- 25 minutes, basting with remaining marinade, or until the inside is no longer pink. High temperatures will cause the marinade to burn.

Root Beer Pork Chops

(Ready in about 2 hours 40 minutes | serving 4|Difficulty: Moderate)

Per serving: Kcal 409, Fat: 9.3g, Net Carbs: 37.5g, Protein: 41.8g

Ingredients

- 4 pork chops, 1 inch thick
- 3 cans root beer, 12 ounces
- Pepper to taste
- Beef stock 1 cup
- Brown sugar 2 tbsp.
- Hot sauce ½ tsp
- Worcestershire sauce 2 tsp
- Salt 1 pinch, to taste

Instructions

1. Put the pork chops in a bowl and cover them with 2 cans of root beer. Refrigerate for at least two hours to marinate. Season the pork chops with pepper and salt after removing them from the root beer.
2. In a saucepan over medium heat, mix the leftover can of root beer, brown sugar, spicy sauce, beef stock, and Worcestershire sauce; simmer until the mixture reduces to approximately 3/4 cup.
3. Preheat an outdoor grill to medium-high heat and brush the grate liberally with oil.
4. Grill the pork chops until they are no longer pink throughout the center, about 6-8 minutes per side, on a hot grill. The temperature should read 145 degrees F on an instant-read thermometer placed into the center. Cook for a further 2 minutes per side after brushing the chops with the reduction sauce. Remove from the grill, then brush with any sauce that has remained. Before serving, season with salt to taste.

Grilled Pork Tenderloin with Balsamic Honey Glaze

(Ready in about 55 minutes | serving 4|Difficulty: Easy)

Per serving: Kcal 251, Fat: 11.8g, Net Carbs: 4.2g, Protein: 30.6g

Ingredients

- Garlic powder 1 tbsp.
- Onion powder 1 tbsp.
- Chili powder 2 tsp
- Paprika 2 tsp
- Salt 1 tsp
- Olive oil 2 tbsp., divided
- 1 pork tenderloin, 3 lbs.
- Balsamic vinegar ¼ cup
- Honey 1 tsp
- Dijon mustard 1 tsp

Instructions

1. Combine the onion, garlic, and chili powders with paprika and salt in a mixing bowl. Rub the pork tenderloin all over with the mixture.

2. Over medium-high heat, heat 1 tbsp. Olive oil. Sear the pork on all sides until golden brown, about 4 minutes per side. The tenderloin should be wrapped in aluminum foil.

3. Preheat an outdoor grill to medium-high heat and brush the grate liberally with oil. Grill the pork for 20 minutes in foil.

4. Meanwhile, whisk together the honey, balsamic vinegar, and mustard with the leftover olive oil. Brush the glaze liberally on all sides of the pork as it is unwrapped on the grill. Continue grilling, spraying on extra glaze as needed, for another 10 minutes or till an instant-read thermometer placed in the center reads 145 degrees F.

5. Allow for a 5-minute rest at room temperature before cutting. If desired, drizzle with any leftover glaze.

Grilled Lemon Herb Pork Chops

(Ready in about 2 hours 25 minutes | serving 4|Difficulty: Moderate)

Per serving: Kcal 203, Fat: 10.1g, Net Carbs: 1.6g, Protein: 25.1g

Ingredients

- Lemon juice ¼ cup
- Vegetable oil 2 tbsp.
- Garlic 4 cloves, minced
- Salt 1 tsp
- Dried oregano ¼ tsp
- Pepper ¼ tsp
- 6 pork loin chops, 4 ounces, boneless

Instructions

1.   Combine garlic, lemon juice, oregano, oil, salt, and pepper in a big resealable bag. Place the chops in a bag, seal them, and place it in the refrigerator for two hours or overnight. To distribute the marinade, turn the bag regularly.

2.   Heat an outdoor grill to high temperatures. Remove the chops from the bag and pour the marinade into a saucepan. Bring the marinade to a boil, then turn off the heat and set it aside.

3.   Grease the grill grate lightly. Grill pork chops for 5 - 6 minutes per side until done, often basting with the boiled marinade.

Grilled Rosemary Pork Chops

(Ready in about 3 hours 20 minutes | serving 4|Difficulty: Moderate)

Per serving: Kcal 273, Fat: 5.8g, Net Carbs: 25.9g, Protein: 29g

Ingredients

- Soy sauce 1 cup
- Water ½ cup
- Brown sugar 6 tbsp.
- Dried rosemary 2 tbsp., crushed
- Pork chops 4 boneless

Instructions

1.   In a mixing bowl, combine the water, soy sauce, brown sugar, and rosemary; pour half of the marinade into the resealable plastic bag. Add the pork chops to the bag, coat them in the marinade, squeeze out excess air, and close it. Refrigerate for at least three hours before serving. Set aside the remaining marinade.

2.   Preheat an outdoor grill to medium heat and brush the grate gently with oil. Remove the pork chops from the marinade and shake off any remaining liquid. Remove the remaining marinade and toss it out.

3.   Place the pork chops on the grill & cook till the pork is no longer pink in the middle, 4 to 5 minutes on each side, occasionally brushing with the remaining marinade. The temperature should read 145 degrees F on an instant-read thermometer placed into the center.

Bada Bing Pork Chops

(Ready in about 8 hours 20 minutes | serving 6|Difficulty: Difficult)
Per serving: Kcal 450, Fat: 22g, Net Carbs: 11.5g, Protein: 49.5g

Ingredients
- Salad dressing 1 cup, Italian-style
- Worcestershire sauce ½ cup
- Applesauce ½ cup
- Hot pepper sauce ¼ cup
- Lime 1, juiced
- 6 pork chops, bone-in

Instructions

1. In a mixing bowl, combine the Worcestershire sauce, Italian dressing, spicy pepper sauce, applesauce, and lime juice. Refrigerate for 6 hours or overnight after pouring the marinade all over the pork chops.

2. Preheat an outdoor grill to medium heat and brush the grate gently with oil.

3. Remove the chops from the marinade and place them in a saucepan with the marinade. Bring the marinade to a boil over a moderate flame, then remove from the heat and set aside for 1 minute. Place the pork chops on the hot grill and cook until thoroughly browned and also no longer pink in the center, about 6 minutes each side, basting the chops with the marinade occasionally. The temperature should read 145 degrees F on an instant-read thermometer placed into the center. Allow the marinade to absorb into the chops completely. Serve.

Molasses Brined Pork Chops

(Ready in about 6 hours 25 minutes | serving 4|Difficulty: Difficult)
Per serving: Kcal 346, Fat: 13.5g, Net Carbs: 31.2g, Protein: 24.5g

Ingredients
- Kosher salt ½ cup
- Molasses ½ cup
- Cloves 4 whole
- Boiling water 1 cup
- Coldwater 7 cups
- 4 pork chops, center cut & bone-in
- Vegetable oil ½ tsp

Instructions

1. In a large bowl, combine the salt, molasses, cloves, and boiling water. Allow cooling to room temperature after stirring until the molasses and salt have dissolved.

2. Pour cold water into the molasses mixture and whisk well.

3. Submerge pork chops completely in molasses mixture. Refrigerate for six hours after covering the bowl.

4. Pat the pork chops dry after removing them from the brine using paper towels. Each chop should be lightly oiled.

5. Preheat an outdoor grill to medium-high heat and brush the grate liberally with oil.

6. Place the pork chops on the hottest portion of the grill and cook for 2 to 3 minutes on each side, or until browned. Transfer the pork to a medium-high portion of the grill and cook for 6 to 8 minutes per side, till it is slightly pink in the center. In the center of the chop, an instant-read thermometer should read 145 degrees F.

Mesquite Grilled Pork Chops with Apple Salsa

(Ready in about 3 hours 28 minutes | serving 4|Difficulty: Moderate)
Per serving: Kcal 384, Fat: 26.7g, Net Carbs: 17.8g, Protein: 18.4g

Ingredients

- 1 jar applesauce, 16 ounce
- Onions 1, quartered
- Jalapeno pepper 1, seeded & minced
- Garlic 1 clove, minced
- Salt ½ tsp
- White pepper 1 tbsp., ground
- Pork chops 4
- Garlic powder 1 ½ tsp
- Pepper & salt to taste
- Mesquite chips 1 cup, soaked

Instructions

1. Combine applesauce, garlic, onion, jalapeño pepper, 1/2 tsp salt, and white pepper in a medium mixing bowl. Refrigerate for at least a few hours or overnight.
2. Salt, Garlic powder, and pepper to taste are used to season the chops.
3. Preheat the grill to medium-high.
4. Place soaked wood on top of the coals or in the smoker box of the gas grill. Place the chops on the grill after lightly oiling the grate. Cook for 6 - 8 minutes per side, or until done to your taste. Serve with a salsa of applesauce.

Swedish Cured Pork Loin

(Ready in about 1 hour 15 minutes | serving 4|Difficulty: Easy)
Per serving: Kcal 277, Fat: 8.2g, Net Carbs: 4.3g, Protein: 43.7g

Ingredients

- Pork loin roast 4 lbs. Boneless
- White sugar 3 tbsp.
- Salt 2 tbsp.
- Cumin 1 tsp, ground
- Cardamom ½ tsp, ground

Instructions

1. Rinse the pork thoroughly and pat it dry. Place it in a big glass dish. Mix the sugar, cumin, salt, and cardamom in a small bowl. Combine all of the ingredients in a large mixing bowl and rub thoroughly over the pork. Refrigerate for 24 - 36 hours after covering.
2. Preheat an outdoor grill on indirect heat and brush the grate gently with oil.
3. Remove the pork from the fridge and toss out any remaining juices. Rinse the meat thoroughly and pat it dry.
4. Grill for about 1 hour over low indirect heat or until the internal temperature of the pork reaches 145°F.

Caribbean-Spiced Pork Tenderloin with Peach Salsa

(Ready in about 35 minutes | serving 4|Difficulty: Easy)

Per serving: Kcal 229, Fat: 11g, Net Carbs: 9g, Protein: 23g

Ingredients

- 3/4 cup fresh peaches, chopped & peeled
- Chopped red pepper 1 small, sweet
- Jalapeno pepper 1, seeded & chopped
- Red onion 2 tbsp., finely chopped
- Cilantro 2 tbsp., minced & fresh
- Lime juice 1 tbsp.
- Garlic clove 1, minced
- Salt 1/8 tsp
- Pepper 1/8 tsp
- Olive oil 2 tbsp.
- Brown sugar 1 tbsp.
- Caribbean jerk seasoning 1 tbsp.
- Thyme 1 tsp, dried
- Rosemary 1 tsp, dried & crushed
- Salt 1/2 tsp, seasoned
- 1 lb. Pork tenderloin

Instructions

1. Blend the first nine ingredients in a small bowl and leave them aside. Mix the oil, jerk spice, brown sugar, thyme, rosemary, and seasoned salt in a separate small bowl. Rub all over the pork.

2. Cover and cook for 9-11 mins over medium heat, till a thermometer reads 145° F. Allow for a 5-minute rest before slicing. Serve with a side of salsa.

Provolone-Stuffed Pork Chops with Tarragon Vinaigrette

(Ready in about 25 minutes | serving 4|Difficulty: Easy)

Per serving: Kcal 702, Fat: 58g, Net Carbs: 3g, Protein: 41g

Ingredients

- Olive oil 1/2 cup
- White balsamic vinegar 1/4 cup
- Fresh tarragon 2 tbsp., minced
- Garlic 2 cloves, minced
- Salt ¼ tsp
- Pepper ¼ tsp
- For pork chops
- 4 pork loin chops, bone-in
- 4 slices cheese
- Olive oil 2 tbsp.
- Minced tarragon 2 tsp, fresh
- Salt ¼ tsp
- Pepper ¼ tsp
- Tomatoes 2 large, each sliced into six wedges

Instructions

1. Whisk together the first 6 ingredients in a small bowl, for serving, set aside 1/4 cup vinaigrette.

2. Cut a pocket in each pork chop by slicing near to the bone, then stuff with cheese. Brush both sides of the chops with a mixture of oil, salt, tarragon, and pepper.

3. Moist a paper towel using cooking oil and rub it on the grill rack with long-handled tongs to lightly coat it. Brush the remaining vinaigrette on the tomato wedges. Grill, uncovered, over medium-high heat for 2-3 mins or until lightly browned, or grill 4 inches from the heat.

4. Grill chops, covered, over medium heat for 5-6 minutes on each side or until a thermometer reads 145° F. Broil chops 4-5 in. from the heat for 4-5 minutes per side or until a thermometer reads 145° F. In the last three minutes of cooking, baste regularly with the leftover vinaigrette. Allow for a 5-minute rest period. Serve with tomatoes and the vinaigrette that was set aside.

(Ready in about 35 minutes | serving 4|Difficulty: Easy)

Per serving: Kcal 300, Fat: 15g, Net Carbs: 9g, Protein: 24g

Ingredients

- Sweet onion 1/2 cup, chopped
- Lime juice 1/2 cup
- Jalapeno peppers 1/4 cup, finely chopped & seeded
- Olive oil 2 tbsp.
- Cumin 4 tsp, ground
- Pork tenderloin 1 ½ lb., sliced into ¾ inch pieces
- Jalapeno pepper jelly 3 tbsp.

For salsa:

- Ripe avocados 2 medium, peeled & chopped
- Cucumber 1 small, seeded & chopped
- Plum tomatoes 2, seeded & chopped
- Onions 2 green, chopped
- 2 tbsp. Cilantro, minced & fresh
- Honey 1 tbsp.
- Salt ¼ tsp
- Pepper ¼ tsp

Instructions

1. To make the marinade, combine the first five ingredients. Mix pork into 1/2 cup marinade in a large mixing bowl; refrigerate for up to 2 hours, covered.

2. In a small saucepan, combine the jelly & 1/3 cup of the leftover marinade; bring to a boil. Cook and whisk for 1-2 minutes, or until slightly thickened; remove from heat. In a large mixing bowl, combine the salsa ingredients and stir lightly with the remaining marinade.

3. Drain the pork and toss out the marinade. Place the pork on a grill rack that has been lightly oiled over medium heat. Grill for 4-5 minutes per side, covered, until a thermometer reaches 145° F, coating with glaze during the last three minutes. Serve with a side of salsa.

Calgary Stampede Ribs

(Ready in about 3 hours | serving 4|Difficulty: Easy)
Per serving: Kcal 394, Fat: 24g, Net Carbs: 21g, Protein: 23g

Ingredients
- Sliced pork baby back ribs 4 lbs.
- Garlic 3 cloves, minced
- Sugar 1 tbsp.
- Salt 2 tsp

- Paprika 1 tbsp.
- Cumin 2 tsp, ground
- Chili powder 2 tsp
- Pepper 2 tsp

For barbecue sauce:
- Butter 2 tbsp.
- Onion 1 small, finely chopped
- Ketchup 1 cup
- Brown sugar 1/4 cup, packed
- Lemon juice 3 tbsp.

- Worcestershire sauce 3 tbsp.
- Cider vinegar 2 tbsp.
- Mustard 1 ½ tsp, ground
- Celery seed 1 tsp
- Cayenne pepper 1/8 tsp

Instructions
1. Preheat the oven to 325 degrees F. Place the ribs in a roasting pan and rub garlic all over them. Cover and bake for about 2 hours, or until the potatoes are soft.
2. Sprinkle salt, sugar, and seasonings over the ribs. Remove from pan and set aside to cool slightly. Refrigerate for 8 hours or overnight, covered.
3. Heat butter in a small skillet over medium heat and sauté onion until soft. Bring the remaining ingredients to a boil, stirring constantly. Reduce heat to low and cook, stirring regularly, until the sauce has thickened, about 10 minutes.
4. Brush some of the sauce on the ribs. Cover and cook for 12-15 minutes over medium heat, flipping and sprinkling with more sauce as needed. Serve with the rest of the sauce.

Flavorful Grilled Pork Tenderloin

(Ready in about 30 minutes | serving 4|Difficulty: Easy)
Per serving: Kcal 135, Fat: 4g, Net Carbs: 1g, Protein: 23g

Ingredients
- Salt 3/4 tsp
- Salt 3/4 tsp
- Poultry seasoning 3/4 tsp
- Onion Powder 3/4 tsp

- Garlic powder 3/4 tsp
- Chili powder 3/4 tsp
- Cayenne pepper 1/8 tsp
- 1 lb. Each pork tenderloins 2

Instructions
1. Seasonings should be mixed and sprinkled over the tenderloins. Cook, covered, at medium heat for 20-25 minutes, till a thermometer reads 145° F, turning once or twice. Allow for a 5-minute rest before slicing.

Doreen's Ham Slices on the Grill

(Ready in about 25 minutes | serving 4|Difficulty: Easy)

Per serving: Kcal 245, Fat: 1.3g, Net Carbs: 58g, Protein: 2.7g

Ingredients

- Brown sugar 1 cup, packed
- Lemon juice ¼ cup
- Prepared horseradish ⅓ cup
- Ham 2 slices

Instructions

1. Preheat an outside grill to high heat and brush the grate gently with oil.
2. Combine lemon juice, brown sugar, and prepared horseradish in a small bowl.
3. Microwave the brown sugar mix for 1 minute on high or until it is heated.
4. Both sides of the ham slices should be scored. Place on the grill that has been preheated. While grilling, often baste with the brown sugar mixture. Grill for 6–8 minutes on each side, or until the desired doneness is reached.

Pork Chops with Dill Pickle Marinade

(Ready in about 8 hours 25 minutes | serving 4|Difficulty: Difficult)

Per serving: Kcal 4, Fat: 0g, Net Carbs: 1.1g, Protein: 0g

Ingredients

- 4 pork chops, center-cut
- Dill pickle juice 1 cup
- Pepper & salt to taste

Instructions

1. In a shallow plate, arrange the pork chops. Pickle juice should be poured over the top. Refrigerate for at least 1 hour, but up to 24 hours is recommended.
2. Preheat an outdoor grill to medium-high heat and brush the grate liberally with oil.
3. Drain the pork chops, then discard out the marinade. Grill the pork chops on the prepared grill for 6 to 8 minutes per side, or till no longer pink in the center. The temperature should read 145 degrees F on an instant-read thermometer placed into the center.

Asian Pork Burger

(Ready in about 30 minutes | serving 4|Difficulty: Easy)

Per serving: Kcal 284, Fat: 16.7g, Net Carbs: 10.5g, Protein: 21.8g

Ingredients

- Pork 2 lbs., ground
- Apple 1 small, peeled & chopped
- Red onion ½, chopped
- Red or green bell pepper ½, chopped
- Teriyaki sauce ¼ cup
- Apple cider ¼ cup
- Ginger 1 teaspoon, ground
- Bread crumbs ½ cup
- Black pepper 1 teaspoon
- Soy sauce 1 teaspoon

Instructions

1. In a mixing bowl, combine the ground pork, onion, apple, bell pepper, apple cider, teriyaki sauce, ground ginger, black pepper, bread crumbs, and soy sauce; shape into four patties. Freeze the patties for 30 minutes before grilling to prevent them from becoming soft.

2. Preheat an outdoor grill to medium-high heat and brush the grate liberally with oil.

3. Cook the burgers on the prepared grill for about 5 minutes per side, until hot, firm, and no longer pink into the center. The temperature should read 160 degrees F on an instant-read thermometer placed into the center.

Mediterranean Grilled Pork Chops

(Ready in about 4 hours 20 minutes | serving 4|Difficulty: Difficult)

Per serving: Kcal 386, Fat: 28.9g, Net Carbs: 1.6g, Protein: 28.3g

Ingredients

- Dried sage 2 tsp, crumbled
- Rosemary leaves, 2 tsp dried & crumbled
- Thyme 1 tsp, dried
- Fennel seed 1 tsp, crushed
- White sugar ½ tsp
- Bay leaf 1, crumbled
- Salt 1 ½ tsp
- 4 pork rib chops, bone-in & ½ inch thick
- ⅓ Cup olive oil, extra-virgin

Instructions

1. Combine the sage, fennel seed, rosemary, sugar, thyme, bay leaf, and salt in a mixing dish and stir well. Rub the herb mixture on both sides of pork chops and drizzle with olive oil. Refrigerate for at least a few hours or overnight.

2. Preheat an outdoor grill to medium heat and brush the grate gently with oil.

3. Grill the chops for about 4 minutes per side, or until they are browned, have nice grill marks, as well as the meat is no longer pink inside. At least 145 degrees F should be read on an instant-read thermometer placed into the thickest portion of a chop.

Grilled Pork Tenderloin with Ginger-Peanut

(Ready in about 8 hours 30 minutes | serving 4|Difficulty: Difficult)

Per serving: Kcal 178, Fat: 7.2g, Net Carbs: 2.7g, Protein: 24.6g

Ingredients

- Fat trimmed 2 pork tenderloins, 16 ounces
- Soy sauce 3 tbsp.
- Sugar 1 ½ tsp
- Sesame oil 1 tbsp.
- Peanut butter 1 tbsp.
- Garlic 1 clove, minced
- Curry powder 1 tsp
- Ginger 1 tbsp., minced & fresh
- Salt ½ tsp

Instructions

1. Fill a big plastic bag halfway with pork. In a mixing bowl, combine sesame oil, soy sauce, sugar, garlic, curry powder, ginger, peanut butter, and salt. Pour the marinade over the tenderloins, seal the bag, and chill overnight.

2. Heat an outdoor grill to high temperatures.

3. Remove any extra marinade from the pork with a paper towel and set it aside at room temperature when the grill heats up. Oil the grill grate lightly. Cook pork for 12 to 15 minutes total, three minutes on each side. When the pork is no longer pink inside and has achieved 145 degrees F, it is ready. Remove the pork from the grill & cover it with a foil tent. Allow 5 minutes for resting before serving.

Tender and juicy Pork loin with honey

(Ready in about 5 hours | serving 3|Difficulty: Difficult)

Per serving: Kcal 302, Fat: 13.6g, Net Carbs: 18.2g, Protein: 24.8g

Ingredients

- Honey 2 tbsp.
- Hoisin sauce 2 tbsp.
- Dark soy sauce 2 tbsp.
- Star anise pod, 1 whole crushed
- Chinese five-spice 1 pinch, powder
- 1 tbsp. Aji mirin, cooking wine
- 1 pork loin roast, boneless

Instructions

1. In a glass measuring cup, mix five-spice powder, honey, dark soy sauce, hoisin sauce, star anise, and aji mirin. Set the microwave oven to 60% power and heat for 22 seconds. Pour the mixture into a big resealable plastic bag after stirring it. Refrigerate pork loin for at least four hours or up to 2 days after adding it to the bag and kneading it to coat it with the marinade.

2. Preheat the grill to medium heat and brush the grate gently with oil.

3. Remove the pork roast from the bag and carefully wrap it in aluminum foil. Remove the marinade that has been used and discard it.

4. Cook for about 50 minutes on a pre-heated grill till an instant-read meat thermometer placed into the thickest part of the roast reaches 155 degrees F Allow 10 minutes for the pork to rest before slicing.

Drunken Ribs

(Ready in about 10 hours 30 minutes | serving 4|Difficulty: Difficult)

Per serving: Kcal 1606, Fat: 92.9g, Net Carbs: 121g, Protein: 40.3g

Ingredients

- Garlic powder 2 ½ tbsp.
- White pepper 1 ½ tbsp.
- Salt 1 ½ tbsp.
- Onion salt 1 tbsp.
- Dried oregano 1 tsp
- Pork spareribs 4 lbs.
- White vinegar ½ cup, distilled
- 12 cans premium lager
- 1 bottle ketchup, 20 ounces
- 1 bottle Worcestershire sauce, 10 ounces
- Maple syrup 1 ½ cups
- Brown sugar 1 cup
- Liquid smoke flavoring 1 cup
- Margarine ½ cup
- Apple cider vinegar ½ cup
- Honey mustard ½ cup

Instructions

1. Combine onion salt, garlic powder, seasoned salt, white pepper, and oregano in a medium mixing bowl.

2. Toss the ribs in a large roasting pan with the garlic powder mix and coat evenly. Pour 1/2 of the beer, which is enough to cover the ribs, into the pan with the distilled white vinegar. Cover the pan and marinate ribs for 8 hours or overnight in the refrigerator.

3. Lightly oil the grill grate and prepare an outdoor grill over indirect, medium heat.

4. Whisk the leftover ketchup, beer, Worcestershire sauce, brown sugar, maple syrup, liquid smoke, apple cider vinegar, margarine, and honey mustard together in a large saucepan. Bring the water to a boil. Cover, lower the heat, and cook for 15 min, till a thick sauce forms.

5. Remove the ribs from the marinade and generously cover them in the sauce. Cook for 1 1/2 to 2 hours on a preheated grill, or until an inner temperature of 160 degrees F is reached while cooking, brush the sauce frequently.

(Ready in about 50 minutes | serving 4|Difficulty: Easy)

Per serving: Kcal 349, Fat: 16g, Net Carbs: 8g, Protein: 11g

Ingredients

- Fresh cilantro 1 cup, chopped & divided
- 1/2 cup shallots, minced & divided
- Lime juice 6 tbsp., fresh & divided
- Vegetable oil 1/4 cup
- Pork tenderloins 2, about 2 ½ lbs.
- Fresh cherries ½ lb.
- Fresno Chile 1 fresh
- Olive oil 1 tbsp., extra-virgin
- Salt & black pepper, to taste

Instructions

1.   Preheat the grill to medium-high. In a resealable plastic bag, mix 1/2 cup cilantro, 4 tbsp. Lime juice, 1/4 cup minced shallots, and vegetable oil. Seal bag and shake to coat pork. Marinate for 15 minutes at room temperature, turning occasionally.

2.   Meanwhile, in a medium mixing bowl, add the leftover 1/2 cup cilantro, 2 tbsp. Lime juice, 1/4 cup shallots, cherries, chile, and olive oil. Season the salsa with a pinch of pepper and salt and leave it aside to let the flavors mix.

3.   Remove the tenderloins from the marinade and season with salt & pepper to taste.

4.   Grill tenderloins for 15 minutes, turning regularly, till a thermometer placed into the meat reads 145°F. Allow 10 minutes to rest. Serve with salsa after cutting into thin slices.

Quick-Brined Grilled Pork Chops with Treviso and Balsamic Glaze

(Ready in about 50 minutes | serving 4|Difficulty: Easy)

Per serving: Kcal 504, Fat: 33g, Net Carbs: 28g, Protein: 24g

Ingredients

- Kosher salt 3 tbsp.
- Sugar 1 1/2 tbsp.
- Pork rib chops 1-inch-thick
- Treviso radicchio 1 head
- Belgian endive 1 head
- Olive oil 3 tbsp., extra-virgin
- Balsamic vinegar 3/4 cup
- Butter 1 tbsp.
- Italian parsley, chopped & fresh

Instructions

1. Prepare the grill (medium-high heat). In an 11 x 7 x 2-inch glass baking dish, combine salt, 1 1/2 cups water, and sugar; mix until salt and sugar are dissolved. Allow pork chops to marinate for 20 minutes, flipping once or twice.

2. Treviso & endive should be quartered lengthwise, with some core attached to each slice. Brush with oil and place on baking sheet. Season to taste with pepper and salt. In a small skillet, reduce the vinegar to 1/4 cup by boiling it for 5 minutes. Add the butter and whisk to combine. Using salt and pepper, season the glaze.

3. Remove the pork from the brine and pat it dry. Brush with oil and season with black pepper. Grill Treviso, pork, and endive for 2 - 3 mins per side for vegetables and 6 - 8 minutes each side for chops until veggies are softened. A thermometer is placed horizontally into the middle of the chops reads 150°F.

4. Place the pork and vegetables on serving dishes. Drizzle glaze over the top and garnish with parsley.

Pork Chops with Fresh Herb Salad (Vietnamese-Style)

(Ready in about 55 minutes | serving 4|Difficulty: Easy)

Per serving: Kcal 277, Fat: 23g, Net Carbs: 28g, Protein: 12g

Ingredients

- Shallot 1 large, chopped
- Garlic 3 cloves, chopped
- Brown sugar 1/3 cup, packed
- Fish sauce 1/4 cup
- Dark soy sauce 2 tbsp.
- Vegetable oil 2 tbsp.
- 2 tsp black pepper, freshly ground
- 4 pork rib chops, bone-in
- Kosher salt
- Red plums 3, sliced into ½ inch wedges
- Scallions 2, thinly sliced
- Fresno Chile 1, thinly sliced
- Cilantro leaves 2 cups
- Bean sprouts 1/2 cup
- Rice vinegar 2 tbsp., unseasoned
- For serving: Lime wedges

Instructions

1. In a blender, combine the shallot, oil, garlic, fish sauce, brown sugar, soy sauce, and pepper. Fill a big resealable plastic bag halfway with marinade. Turn the pork chop to coat it with the sauce. Refrigerate for at least one hour or up to 12 hours after sealing the bag and pressing out the air.

2. Preheat the grill to medium-high. Remove the pork chops, allowing the excess to drop back into the bag of marinade, and season all sides with salt. Place pork chops on the grill for 2 minutes per side, rotating once, until seared.

3. In a large mixing bowl, combine the bean sprouts, plums, Chile, scallions, herbs, and vinegar. Season with salt and toss once more.

4. Pork should be served with lime wedges and salad.

PART 2: POULTRY RECIPES

BBQ Grilled Chicken

(Ready in about 30 minutes | serving 4|Difficulty: Easy)

Per serving: Kcal 226, Fat: 15g, Net Carbs: 0.1g, Protein: 23g

Ingredients

- Barbecue sauce 2 cups
- 1 lime juice
- Honey 2 tbsp.
- Hot sauce 1 tbsp.
- Kosher salt
- Black pepper, freshly ground
- 1 pound chicken breasts, boneless & skinless
- For grill, vegetable oil

Instructions

1. Combine lime juice, barbecue sauce, honey, and spicy sauce in a large mixing bowl and season with pepper and salt. Set aside 1/2 cup of the liquid for basting.
2. Toss the chicken in the bowl until it is well coated.
3. Preheat the grill to high heat. Grill chicken till charred, 8 minutes each side for breasts and 10- 12 minutes each side for drumsticks, basting with remaining marinade.

Grilled Pineapple Chicken

(Ready in about 25 minutes | serving 4|Difficulty: Easy)

Per serving: Kcal 240, Fat: 1.6g, Net Carbs: 18.7g, Protein: 35.7g

Ingredients

- Pineapple juice 1 cup, unsweetened
- Ketchup ¾ cup
- Soy sauce ½ cup, low sodium
- Brown sugar ½ cup
- Garlic 2 cloves, minced
- 1 tbsp. Ginger, freshly minced
- 1 lb. Chicken breasts, boneless & skinless
- Vegetable oil 1 tsp.
- Pineapple 1, sliced into halved
- Green onions thinly sliced for garnish

Instructions

1. Whisk together garlic, ketchup, soy sauce, pineapple juice, brown sugar, and ginger in a large mixing bowl until well blended.
2. Pour the marinade over the chicken in a big resealable plastic bag. Allow at least two hours or up to overnight to marinate in the fridge.
3. Preheat the grill to high when you're ready to cook. Grill the chicken, basting it with the marinade until it's browned and cooked through, about 8 minutes per side.
4. Cover pineapple with oil, then place on grill for 2 minutes per side, or until charred.
5. Before serving, garnish the pineapple and chicken with green onions.

Grilled Chicken Wings

(Ready in about 35 minutes | serving 4|Difficulty: Easy)
Per serving: Kcal 284, Fat: 6.2g, Net Carbs: 0g, Protein: 53.4g

Ingredients

For wings

- 1 Lemon zest
- Kosher salt 2 tsp.
- Smoked paprika 1 tsp.
- Garlic powder 1 tsp.
- Onion powder 1 tsp.
- Dried thyme 1 tsp.
- Cayenne 1/4 tsp.
- Chicken wings 2 pounds
- For grill, vegetable oil

For sauce

- Mayonnaise 1/2 cup
- 1/2 lemon juice
- Dijon mustard 1 tbsp.
- Horseradish 2 tsp.
- Chives 2 tsp. , freshly chopped
- Hot sauce 1 tsp. , such as Crystal

Instructions

1.   To make the wings, combine lemon zest, paprika, salt, garlic powder, thyme, onion powder, and cayenne in a medium mixing bowl. Place the chicken wings in a large mixing bowl after patting them dry. Toss in the spice mixture to coat.

2.   Preheat the grill to medium. Vegetable oil should be used to coat the grill grates. Cook, occasionally stirring, for 15 - 20 minutes, or until the skin is crisp and the chicken is cooked through.

3.   Meanwhile, prepare the sauce: Whisk together mayonnaise, mustard, horseradish, lemon juice, chives, and spicy sauce in a medium mixing bowl.

4.   Serve the wings with a dipping sauce while they're still hot.

Sweet Chili-Lime Grilled Chicken

(Ready in about 25 minutes | serving 4|Difficulty: Easy)
Per serving: Kcal 247, Fat: 7g, Net Carbs: 18g, Protein: 27g

Ingredients

- Sweet chili sauce ¾ cup
- 2 lime juice
- 1/3 cup soy sauce, low sodium
- 4 chicken breasts, boneless & skinless
- For grill, vegetable oil
- Green onions, thinly sliced, for garnish
- For serving, lime wedges

Instructions

1.   Whisk together the lime juice, chili sauce, and soy sauce in a large mixing bowl. Set aside a quarter-cup of the marinade.

2.   Pour the marinade over the chicken in a big resealable plastic bag. Allow at least two hours or up to overnight to marinate in the fridge.

3.   Preheat the grill to high when you're ready to cook. Grill chicken until blackened and cooked throughout, about 6-8 minutes per side, brushing with marinade.

4.   Serve with a brushing of the reserved marinade and a sprinkling of green onions. Garnish with lime wedges on the side.

Copycat Chipotle Chicken

(Ready in about 35 minutes | serving 4|Difficulty: Easy)
Per serving: Kcal 293, Fat: 18.7g, Net Carbs: 5.8g, Protein: 24.9g

Ingredients
For chicken

- Red onion 1/2, chopped
- Garlic 2 cloves
- Chipotle pepper 1 in adobo sauce
- Chipotle sauce 1 tbsp.
- Vegetable oil 3 tbsp.
- 1 lime juice

For bowls

- Cooked Rice
- Black beans
- Corn

- Oregano 1 tsp. , dried
- Cumin 1/2 tsp., ground
- Kosher salt
- Black pepper, freshly ground
- 1 lb. Chicken breasts, boneless & skinless

- Guacamole
- Lime wedges
- Salsa

Instructions

1. Blend garlic, onion, adobo sauce and chipotle pepper, oil, oregano, lime juice, and cumin till smooth in a food processor. Using salt and pepper, season to taste.
2. In a big resealable plastic bag, combine the marinade and the chicken and rub all over to coat. Allow at least two hours in the fridge to marinate.
3. Preheat the grill to high and bring the chicken to room temperature. Remove the chicken from the marinade and toss it out. Grill the chicken for about 8 minutes per side, or until it is cooked through and the internal temperature reaches 165° F.
4. Serve the chicken with rice.

Chicken, Tomatoes, and Corn Foil Packs

(Ready in about 30 minutes | serving 4|Difficulty: Easy)
Per serving: Kcal 277, Fat: 23g, Net Carbs: 28g, Protein: 12g

Ingredients

- 4 chicken breasts, boneless & skinless
- Grape tomatoes 2 cups, halved
- Corn 2 ears, kernels stripped
- Garlic 2 cloves, thinly sliced
- 1/4 cup olive oil, extra-virgin

- Butter 2 tbsp.
- Kosher salt
- Black pepper, freshly ground
- For garnish, fresh basil

Instructions

1. Preheat the grill to high heat. Cut four 12" long sheets of foil. Add a chicken breast, corn, tomatoes, and garlic to each sheet of foil. Sprinkle each with oil and a piece of butter on top. Using salt and pepper, season to taste.
2. Fold the foil packages in half crosswise over the chicken and close the top and bottom edges.
3. Grill for 15 to 20 minutes, or till fully cooked through or vegetables are soft.
4. Serve with basil on top.

Honey Balsamic Grilled Chicken Thighs

(Ready in about 1 hour 25 minutes | serving 6|Difficulty: Easy)

Per serving: Kcal 380, Fat: 24.7g, Net Carbs: 13.3g, Protein: 25.5g

Ingredients

- 8 chicken thighs, bone-in & skin-on
- Kosher salt
- Black pepper, freshly ground
- Butter 2 tbsp.
- Balsamic vinegar 2 tbsp.
- Honey 1/3 cup
- Garlic 3 cloves, peeled & crushed
- For oiling, canola oil
- For garnish: chopped chives, lemon wedges, chopped parsley

Instructions

1. Sprinkle pepper and salt on all sides of the chicken thighs on a big plate. Using your hands, rub the spices into the chicken. Allow cooling for at least an hour in the refrigerator.

2. In the meantime, make the glaze: Melt the butter in a medium saucepan. Stir in the honey, vinegar, and garlic until the honey is completely dissolved. Using salt and pepper, season to taste.

3. Preheat the grill to medium and brush the grates using canola oil. Add the chicken skin side down to the grill and cook for 10 minutes per side, flipping frequently and basting with sauce.

4. Serve with lemon wedges, chives and parsley on the side.

Jamaican Jerk Chicken

(Ready in about 40 minutes | serving 4|Difficulty: Easy)

Per serving: Kcal 495, Fat: 25g, Net Carbs: 51g, Protein: 17g

Ingredients

- 2 lbs. Chicken breasts, skinless
- Jalapeno pepper 1, seeded & diced
- 3 tbsp. Water
- 1 lime juice
- 1 lemon juice
- Dijon mustard 1 tbsp.
- Garlic 2 cloves, minced
- Chicken bouillon 2 cubes
- Parsley 1 tsp, dried
- Cumin 1 tsp, ground
- Thyme ½ tsp, dried
- Cinnamon ½ tsp
- Black pepper ½ tsp
- Cinnamon 1 dash

Instructions

1. In a small resealable plastic bag, mix all ingredients except the chicken. Add in the chicken and toss to coat.

2. Cover and refrigerate for 30 minutes to marinate in jerk seasoning. Preheat the grill to high. Remove the chicken from the jerk marinade and place it in a saucepan.

3. Bring the water to a boil. Place the chicken on the grill and cook for 7- 10 minutes per side, basting with the leftover jerk marinade.

Mediterranean Chicken Salad

(Ready in about 1 hour 25 minutes | serving 4|Difficulty: Easy)

Per serving: Kcal 284.6, Fat: 8.3g, Net Carbs: 22.6g, Protein: 30.4g

Ingredients

For the Dressing

- Olive oil 1/2 cup
- Lemon juice 1/4 cup
- Oregano 1 tbsp. Dried
- Salt 1/2 tsp
- Black pepper 1/4 tsp, ground

For the Salad

- 4 chicken breasts, skinless & boneless
- Baby spinach 2 cups
- Red onion ½, peeled &thinly sliced
- Halved cherry tomatoes, 2 cups
- Pitted & halved black olives 1/2 cup
- Feta cheese 1/2 cup
- Pita bread 4

Instructions

Gather the ingredients.

1. Whisk together half a cup of olive oil, dried oregano, a half cup of lemon juice, salt, and powdered black pepper in a large mixing bowl.

2. Half of the mixture should be kept in a separate small bowl for dressing. Add the leftover half of the marinade to the chicken breasts and coat them completely. Refrigerate for roughly one hour, but no longer than four hours, covered in plastic wrap.

3. Preheat an outdoor grill to 400 degrees F.

4. Cook for 5 minutes on one side, then flip and cook for another 5 minutes, or until the chicken is cooked completely and no longer pink.

5. Cut the chicken in half lengthwise.

6. Toss the baby spinach and other salad greens, chopped red onion, cherry tomatoes, olives, and feta cheese in a separate bowl. Toss all together with the dressing.

7. Place the salad on a plate and top with grilled chicken slices & toasted pita bread.

(Ready in about 1 hour 25 minutes | serving 4|Difficulty: Easy)

Per serving: Kcal 276, Fat: 13g, Net Carbs: 24g, Protein: 17g

Ingredients

- 4 skinless chicken breasts (6 ounces each), boneless & skinless

For the Marinade

- Soy sauce 1/2 cup
- Garlic 3 cloves, peeled & crushed
- Rice wine vinegar 1/4 cup
- Honey 2 tbsp.
- Ginger root 1 tbsp., fresh, peeled & grated
- Chopped green onions 4 medium
- 2 tbsp. Sesame oil, toasted
- 1 tsp sesame seeds, toasted
- Garnish: cilantro leaves 2 tbsp., fresh

Instructions

1. To make the marinade, put the soy sauce, vinegar, garlic, honey, onions, ginger, sesame oil, & sesame seeds in a big plastic zip-top bag.

2. Seal the bag tightly after adding the chicken breasts and pressing out any excess air. Refrigerate for 30 - 60 minutes after removing the bag from the fridge.

3. Remove the chicken from the refrigerator twenty minutes before you plan to cook it. Coat a grill grates with a thin layer of cooking oil and heat to high.

4. Remove the chicken from the marinade and set it aside. 6 mins per side on the grill until completely cooked and tender. Serve with cilantro leaves as a garnish.

Grilled chicken stuffed with cheese and peppers

(Ready in about 30 minutes | serving 4|Difficulty: Easy)

Per serving: Kcal 501, Fat: 20.5g, Net Carbs: 38.2g, Protein: 39.1g

Ingredients

- Chicken breast 4, boneless & skinless
- Sweet peppers 8, sliced
- Pepper jack cheese 4 slices
- Colby jack cheese 4 slices
- Creole seasoning 1 tbsp.
- Black pepper 1 tsp
- Garlic powder 1 tsp
- Onion powder 1 tsp
- Olive oil, extra-virgin
- Toothpicks

Instructions

1. Rinse and pat dry the chicken.
2. Combine the seasonings and set them aside.
3. Cut a slit down the length of each chicken breast, but don't cut all the way through.
4. Rub olive oil all over the outside and inside of the chicken.
5. Season both sides of the chicken as well as the inside of the slit with the spice blend.
6. Slice the peppers into the rings and half the cheese.
7. Place a slice of cheese on the bottom of the chicken, top with peppers, and another slice of cheese.
8. 3–4 toothpicks are used to secure the chicken.
9. Grill the chicken for Eight minutes per side on a hot grill. Alternatively, cook until the chicken reaches an internal temperature of 165 degrees F.
10. Allow time for the chicken to rest before removing the toothpicks and serving.

Grilled honey lime cilantro chicken

(Ready in about 15 minutes | serving 4|Difficulty: Easy)

Per serving: Kcal 314, Fat: 9g, Net Carbs: 25g, Protein: 35g

Ingredients

- Chicken breasts 2 lbs., boneless & skinless
- Lime juice 1/4 cup
- Honey 1/2 cup
- Soy Sauce 2 tbsp.
- Olive oil 1 tbsp.
- Minced garlic 2 cloves
- Cilantro 1/2 cup, finely chopped
- Salt 1/2 tsp
- Pepper 1/4 tsp

Instructions

1. Combine honey, lime juice, soy sauce, garlic, olive oil, cilantro, salt, and pepper in a small bowl.
2. Let the chicken marinate in the sauce for 3-4 hours or overnight.
3. Preheat the grill to a medium-high temperature. Grill the chicken for 3-4 minutes on each side, or till cooked through and no longer pink.

(Ready in about 30 minutes | serving 4|Difficulty: Easy)

Per serving: Kcal 181, Fat: 8g, Net Carbs: 15g, Protein: 20g

Ingredients

- 4 chicken breasts, boneless & skinless, sliced into large cubes
- Honey ¼ cup
- Soy sauce 4 tbsp.
- Olive oil 2 tsp, plus extra for grill
- Garlic 2 cloves, minced
- Sriracha Chile 3 tbsp. Sauce
- Salt ¼ tsp
- 4 skewers

Instructions

1. Set aside the chicken cubes in a large zip lock bag.
2. Whisk together honey, sriracha, olive oil, soy sauce, garlic, and salt in a small bowl.
3. Divide the mixture, reserving 1/4 cup for later use.
4. Pour the remaining mixture into the bag with the chicken, squeeze out the air, seal the bag, coat the chicken in sauce, and marinate for at least 30 minutes.
5. Preheat the grill to medium/high. Add 4-6 chicken pieces per skewer using soaked wood or metal skewers; repeat until all chicken is skewered. Remove the marinade that has been used and discard it.
6. Brush oil onto the grill grates using a grill brush to prevent sticking; alternatively, use grill spray. Close the grill after placing the skewers on it. Grill the chicken over medium-high heat, brushing it with the leftover sauce mixture now and then. Between regular brushing, close the grill. Cook for 5-6 minutes on the first side, then flip and cook for another 4-5 minutes.
7. Serve immediately and enjoy.

Thai Lemongrass Grilled Chicken

(Ready in about 2 hours 30 minutes | serving 4|Difficulty: Moderate)
Per serving: Kcal 240, Fat: 7g, Net Carbs: 3g, Protein: 39g
Ingredients

- Chicken thighs 4-6
- Lemongrass 2 stalks
- 1/2 lime juice
- Fish sauce 3 tbsp.
- Soy sauce 1 tbsp.

- Brown sugar 2 1/2 tbsp.
- Finely chopped onion 1/4 cup
- Minced garlic 4 cloves
- Red chilies 2 fresh

Instructions

1. Open up chicken thighs & place them flat in a baking dish, preferably one with a flat bottom.
2. Remove the bulb end of each lemongrass stalk before slicing the rest. Remove the upper stem and discard it. Pulse it in a food processor until it forms a fragrant, watery paste. Mix it with soy sauce, fish sauce, and brown sugar to prepare the marinade paste.
3. Spread the paste over the chicken, turning it to coat each piece. Spoon the garlic, onions, and chilies onto the chicken's tops with a spoon.
4. Cover then marinate for at least 2 hours, but up to 6 hours.
5. Spray a hot grill with just a little vegetable oil before grilling the chicken until it's cooked through.
6. Serve the chicken with a side of a salad, and you're ready to go.

Grilled Chicken Parmesan

(Ready in about 20 minutes | serving 4|Difficulty: Easy)
Per serving: Kcal 331, Fat: 8g, Net Carbs: 42g, Protein: 22g

Ingredients

- Chicken breasts 4, skinless & boneless
- Roma tomatoes 3, sliced thinly
- 4 ounces mozzarella cheese
- Parmesan cheese 1/4 cup

- Basil leaves 6
- Olive oil 2 tsp
- Salt 1/2 tsp
- Black pepper 1/2 tsp

Instructions

1. Preheat the grill to medium-high.
2. Pounded the chicken breasts to a thickness of about 1/4 inch.
3. Using salt, olive oil, and black pepper, coat the chicken.
4. Cook the chicken for 5 minutes on the grill.
5. Place tomato slices and cheese on top of the chicken.
6. Cook for a total of 6 - 8 minutes.
7. Remove the chicken from the heat when the internal temperature reaches 165 degrees F, set aside for 1 to 2 minutes, then garnish with basil leaves before serving.
8. Make a chicken parmesan sandwich or serve over pasta.

Eastern Grilled Chicken Breasts

(Ready in about 1 hour 25 minutes | serving 4|Difficulty: Easy)
Per serving: Kcal 276, Fat: 13g, Net Carbs: 24g, Protein: 17g

Ingredients

- 4 chicken breasts, boneless & skinless
- For the marinade
- Soy sauce 1/2 cup
- Peeled & crushed garlic 3 cloves
- Rice wine vinegar 1/4 cup
- Honey 2 tbsp.
- Peeled & grated ginger root 1 tbsp., fresh
- Chopped green onions 4 medium
- Sesame oil 2 tbsp.
- Sesame seeds 1 tsp
- For Garnish 2 tbsp. Cilantro leaves, whole fresh

Instructions

1. To prepare the marinade, combine the garlic, soy sauce, sesame oil, vinegar, ginger, honey, onions, and sesame seeds in a big plastic zip-top bag.
2. Seal the bag tightly after adding the chicken breasts and pressing out any excess air. Refrigerate for 30- 60 minutes after removing the bag from the fridge.
3. Remove the chicken from the refrigerator twenty minutes before you plan to cook it. Coat a grill with a thin layer of cooking oil and heat to high.
4. Remove the chicken from the marinade and set it aside. Cook for 6 minutes per side on the grill or until completely cooked and tender. Serve with cilantro leaves as a garnish.

Pineapple Salsa Grilled Chicken

(Ready in about 2 hours 25 minutes | serving 4|Difficulty: Moderate)
Per serving: Kcal 274, Fat: 7.7g, Net Carbs: 13.9g, Protein: 36g

Ingredients

- 4 limes juice, divided
- 1/4 cup+ 1 tbsp. Cilantro, freshly chopped
- 1/4 cup olive oil, extra-virgin plus more for the grill
- Honey 2 tsp.
- Kosher salt
- 1 lb. Chicken breasts, boneless & skinless
- Pineapple 2 cups, chopped
- 1 diced avocado
- Red onion 1/4, diced
- Black pepper freshly ground

Instructions

1. To make the marinade, follow these steps: Combine the juice of 3 limes, oil, 1/4 cup cilantro, and honey in a large mixing bowl and season with salt.
2. Pour the marinade over the chicken in a big resealable plastic bag. Allow at least two hours, or up to overnight, to marinate in the refrigerator.
3. Preheat the grill to high when you're ready to cook. Grill chicken till charred and cooked throughout, about 8 minutes per side, on oiled grill grates.
4. Meanwhile, combine pineapple, red onion, avocado, remaining lime juice, and cilantro in a medium mixing bowl. Using salt and pepper, season to taste.
5. Before serving, spoon salsa over the chicken.

Bruschetta Grilled Chicken

(Ready in about 50 minutes | serving 4|Difficulty: Easy)
Per serving: Kcal 282, Fat: 11g, Net Carbs: 7g, Protein: 38.5g

Ingredients

- 4 tbsp. Olive oil, extra-virgin
- 1 lemon juice, divided
- Kosher salt
- Black pepper, freshly ground
- 1 tsp. Dried oregano
- 4 chicken breasts, boneless & skinless
- Tomatoes 3 slices, chopped
- Garlic 2 cloves, minced
- Basil 1 tbsp., freshly chopped
- Mozzarella 4 slices
- Parmesan freshly grated, for serving

Instructions

1. In a small mixing bowl, whisk together the oil, half of the 1/4 tsp pepper, lemon juice, 1 tsp salt, and Italian seasoning. Refrigerate for thirty min after transferring to a big resealable bag with chicken.
2. Heat the grill to medium-high heat before adding the chicken and removing the leftover marinade. Grill for 5 to 7 minutes per side on the grill until blackened and cooked to an internal temperature of 165° F.
3. In the meantime, season tomatoes, basil, garlic, and lemon juice with salt and pepper. While the chicken is still on the grill, topped each breast with 1 mozzarella slice and cover for 2 to 3 minutes, or until the cheese is melted. Toss the tomato mixture on top of the chicken.
4. Serve with a sprinkle of Parmesan cheese on top.

California Grilled Chicken

(Ready in about 40 minutes | serving 4|Difficulty: Easy)
Per serving: Kcal 415, Fat: 18g, Net Carbs: 26.9g, Protein: 41.4g

Ingredients

- Balsamic vinegar 3/4 cup
- Garlic powder 1 tsp.
- Honey 2 tbsp.
- Olive oil 2 tbsp., extra-virgin
- Italian seasoning, 2 tsp.
- Kosher salt
- Black pepper, freshly ground
- 4 chicken breasts, boneless & skinless
- Mozzarella 4 slices
- Tomato 4 slices
- Avocado 4 slices
- 2 tbsp. Basil, freshly sliced for garnish
- For drizzling balsamic glaze

Instructions

1. Season with pepper and salt and whisk together garlic powder, oil, balsamic vinegar, honey, and Italian seasoning in a small bowl. Pour over the chicken and set aside for 20 minutes to marinate.
2. Preheat the grill to medium-high when you're ready to cook. Grill chicken till charred & cooked through, about 8 minutes per side, on oiled grill grates.
3. Cover the grill for 2 minutes to melt the avocado, mozzarella, and tomato on top of the chicken.
4. Sprinkle with balsamic glaze and garnish with basil.

Pat's Beer Can Grilled Chicken

(Ready in about 1 hour 50 minutes | serving 4|Difficulty: Easy)
Per serving: Kcal 291, Fat: 11g, Net Carbs: 2g, Protein: 40g

Ingredients

For Chicken Rub

- Smoked paprika 2 tbsp.
- Salt 2 tbsp.
- Onion powder 2 tbsp.
- Cayenne pepper 1 tbsp.
- Cumin 1 tbsp., ground
- Thyme 2 tsp, dried
- Oregano 2 tsp, dried
- Black pepper 2 tsp
- Garlic powder 2 tsp

For the Chicken

- Chicken 4 lbs., washed & dried
- 1 can beer, 12 ounces
- Vegetable oil

Instructions

1. To make the chicken rub, combine all of the ingredients in a medium bowl and use grilled chicken. Extra rub mixture can be kept in an airtight jar for up to six months.
2. For the chicken, prepare as follows: Preheat the grill to medium-high temperature.
3. Add the vegetable oil to the chicken as well as its cavities. Coat the chicken with the rub mixture, making sure to coat the cavity as well. 1/4 of the beer should be poured out, and the chicken should be placed on top of the beer can. Cover the chicken and place it in the middle of the heated grill. Cook the chicken for 1-1 1/2 hrs. Or until it reaches 165 degrees F on an instant-read thermometer. Cover loosely using foil after cooking and set aside for ten minutes before carving.

Tequila Lime Chicken

(Ready in about 8 hours 30 minutes | serving 4|Difficulty: Difficult)
Per serving: Kcal 277, Fat: 14g, Net Carbs: 4g, Protein: 31g

Ingredients

- Gold tequila 1/2 cup
- 1 cup lime juice
- 1/2 cup orange juice
- Chili powder 1 tbsp.
- Minced jalapeno pepper 1 tbsp.
- Minced garlic 1 tbsp.
- Kosher salt 2 tsp
- 1 tsp black pepper, freshly ground
- Chicken breasts 3 whole, skin on & boneless

Instructions

1. In a medium mixing bowl, combine the orange juice, jalapeño pepper, lime juice, chili powder, tequila, pepper, garlic, and salt. Add chicken breasts into it. Refrigerate for at least one night.
2. To keep the chicken from sticking, heat a grill using coals and coat the rack with oil. Remove your chicken breasts from marinade, season generously with pepper and salt, and grill skin-side down for 5 minutes, or until thoroughly browned. Cook for the next 10 minutes, or until the chicken is just cooked through. Transfer to a platter after removing from the grill. Allow for a 5-minute rest period after covering tightly. Serve at room temperature or hot.

Grilled BBQ Lime Chicken

(Ready in about 2 hours 30 minutes | serving 6|Difficulty: Moderate)
Per serving: Kcal 250, Fat: 9g, Net Carbs: 6g, Protein: 32g

Ingredients

- 1 lb. Chicken breasts, boneless & skinless
- Water 2 cup
- Kosher salt 2 tbsp.
- Brown sugar 1/4 cup, packed
- Kosher salt
- Black pepper, freshly ground
- Barbecue sauce 1 cup
- Lime 2, freshly squeezed
- Garlic 2 cloves, minced

Instructions

1. Pound the chicken in a big Ziploc bag until it is 1/4" thick. Whisk together salt, water, and sugar in a large mixing bowl until well blended. Fill a Ziploc bag with brine and chill for at least fifteen minutes, but preferably two hours.
2. Remove the chicken from the brine and discard the liquid.
3. Preheat the grill to medium heat. Season the chicken with pepper and salt, then grill for 6 minutes on each side.
4. Whisk together the lime juice, barbecue sauce, and garlic in a medium mixing bowl. Cook until the chicken is caramelized and cooked through, flipping occasionally.

San Francisco Grilled Chicken Sandwiches

(Ready in about 20 minutes | serving 4|Difficulty: Easy)
Per serving: Kcal 565, Fat: 28g, Net Carbs: 36g, Protein: 63g

Ingredients

- 2 halves of chicken breast, boneless & skinless
- Italian salad dressing 3 tbsp.
- Muenster cheese, 2 slices
- Kaiser rolls 2
- Spinach leaves 8
- Alfalfa sprouts 1/2 cup
- Avocado 6 slices
- Salsa (chunky-style) 2 tbsp.

Instructions

1. Pound chicken breast pieces to a thickness of 1/4 inch. Pour dressing over the chicken in a small bowl. Refrigerate 1 hour after covering and marinating.
2. Chicken should be drained, and the dressing should be discarded. Grill for 3 minutes on medium coals, then flip. Place a cheddar slice on top of each chicken breast half and grill for another 2 minutes or until the chicken is cooked throughout. Half of the sprouts, spinach leaves, and avocado slices should go on the bottom half of each roll. Grilled chicken breast, half of the salsa, and the top half of the bun go on top of each sandwich.

Ginger Grilled Chicken Satay

(Ready in about 2 hours 35 minutes | serving 4|Difficulty: Moderate)
Per serving: Kcal 264, Fat: 2.8g, Net Carbs: 34g, Protein: 26g

Ingredients
- 1 lb. Chicken tenders
- Soy sauce ½ cup
- Brown sugar ½ cup
- 2 tbsp. Ginger, freshly grated
- Fish sauce, 2 tsp
- Lime 1, juiced
- Thin skewers 16, metal
- Cornstarch 1 tbsp.
- Scallion 1, chopped

Instructions
1. To get thin slices, cut the chicken in half lengthwise. To help tenderize the meat, lightly prick it with a fork or even a knife.
2. In a large mixing bowl or resealable plastic bag, mix soy sauce, fish sauce, ginger, brown sugar, and lime juice. Add the chicken tenders and make sure they are completely covered in the marinade. Refrigerate for at least two hours after covering with plastic wrap.
3. Preheat an outdoor grill to high heat and brush the grate gently with oil. Remove the chicken from the marinade and thread it onto skewers made of metal.
4. Meanwhile, combine the marinade and cornstarch in a small saucepan and bring to a boil. Boil for 3 to 4 minutes or until the sauce has thickened. Remove sauce from heat and place in a medium bowl for dipping.
5. Grill skewers until no longer pink into the center, about five minutes per side, on a prepared grill. Serve with a scallion garnish and a side of sauce.

Grilled Chicken with Spinach and Pine Nut Pesto

(Ready in about 25 minutes | serving 4|Difficulty: Easy)
Per serving: Kcal 419, Fat: 32g, Net Carbs: 3g, Protein: 31g

Ingredients
- 2 chicken breasts, boneless
- 2 cups baby spinach leaves, lightly packed
- Pine nuts 1/4 cup, toasted
- Lemon juice, 2 tbsp. Fresh
- Lemon peel 2 tsp, grated
- Olive oil 1/3 cup + 2 tsp
- Salt & black pepper
- 1/3 cup parmesan, freshly grated

Instructions
1. Preheat a grill to medium-high temperature. Oil the grill with a little coating of oil. Using salt and pepper, season the chicken. Grill for five minutes per side on the grill until chicken is cooked through.
2. In a food processor, mix the spinach, lemon juice, pine nuts, and peel. Pulse lightly. Blend in 1/3 cup of oil until the mixture is creamy while the machine is running. Add salt to it. Fill ice cube trays halfway with pesto and freeze for later use.
3. In a medium mixing dish, place the remaining spinach mixture. Mix the Parmesan and the rest of the ingredients in a large mixing bowl. Add salt and pepper to taste the pesto.
4. Serve each piece of chicken with a dollop of pesto on top.

Grilled Chicken with Salsa Verde

(Ready in about 40 minutes | serving 4|Difficulty: Easy)

Per serving: Kcal 247, Fat: 6.2g, Net Carbs: 11.5g, Protein: 40.2g

Ingredients

- For grill grates, vegetable oil
- Lime juice, 1/4 cup fresh
- Garlic 3 cloves, sliced
- Chipotle Chile 1 in adobo, chopped
- Kosher salt & black pepper
- 2 large chicken breasts, boneless & skinless
- Tomatillos 1 lb., husked & rinsed
- Jalapeno 1/4
- Onion 1/4 medium
- Cilantro 4 sprigs, fresh
- Tortillas, for serving

Instructions

1. Preheat an outdoor grill. For at least 30 minutes, soak 4 (12-inch) wooden skewers in water.

2. In a medium bowl, mix the 2 garlic cloves, lime juice, and chipotle. Using salt and pepper, season to taste. Toss in the chicken, tossing well to coat, then set aside to marinate for 20 minutes.

3. Meanwhile, cover the tomatillos with water in a medium saucepan. Bring to a boil, then reduce to low heat and cook until cooked, about 7 minutes. Drain. In a blender, blend the jalapeno, onion, remaining 1 garlic clove, onion, and 1 teaspoon salt until smooth. Puree the cooked tomatillos with the cilantro sprigs until smooth.

4. Remove the chicken from the marinade and thread it onto the skewers that have been soaked in water. Oil your grill grates lightly. Cook for 4 to 6 minutes on the grill, frequently rotating until the chicken is cooked through. Serve warm tortillas with salsa.

Grilled Chicken with Basil Dressing

(Ready in about 1 hour 6 minutes | serving 4|Difficulty: Easy)

Per serving: Kcal 487, Fat: 33.6g, Net Carbs: 2g, Protein: 47.5g

Ingredients

- 2/3 cup olive oil, extra-virgin
- Lemon juice, 3 tbsp. Plus 1/4 cup
- Fennel seeds 1 1/2 tsp, coarsely crushed
- Salt 1 1/2 tsp
- 1 tsp black pepper, freshly ground
- 3 chicken thighs, bone-in, & skin-on
- 3 chicken breasts, bone-in & skin-on
- 1 cup basil leaves, lightly packed
- Garlic clove 1 large
- Lemon peel 1 tsp, grated

Instructions

1.   In a resealable plastic bag, mix fennel seeds, 1/3 cup oil, 3 tbsp. Lemon juice, 3/4 tsp salt, and 1/2 tsp pepper. Seal the bag after adding the chicken. The chicken should be rubbed with the marinade. Refrigerate the chicken for at least 30 min and up to a day, turning it occasionally.

2.   Meanwhile, in a blender, combine the basil, lemon peel, 1/4 cup lemon juice, garlic, 3/4 tsp salt, and 1/2 tsp pepper until smooth. Blend in the leftover 1/3 cup oil gradually. If desired, season the basil sauce with extra salt and pepper to taste.

3.   Preheat the grill at medium-high heat. Remove the chicken from the marinade and set it aside. Discard the marinade and grill the chicken for about Eight minutes per side, or until it is just cooked through. Serve the chicken on serving plates with the basil sauce drizzled on top.

Maple-Brined Grilled Chicken

(Ready in about 3 hours 25 minutes | serving 4|Difficulty: Moderate)

Per serving: Kcal 156, Fat: 4g, Net Carbs: 3g, Protein: 27g

Ingredients

- Maple syrup, 1 tbsp. Pure
- Garlic 3 cloves, smashed
- Thyme sprigs small bunch, fresh
- Kosher salt & black pepper
- 2 lbs. Chicken pieces, bone-in (such as thighs, legs, & breasts)
- For grill, vegetable oil or olive
- For serving: cornbread, green salad

Instructions

1.   In a large mixing bowl, whisk together the garlic, maple syrup, thyme, 1 tbsp. Salt, a generous pinch of pepper, and 3 cups water till the salt is dissolved. Place the chicken in the brine, making sure it is well covered. Put it in the fridge for 2 - 3 hours, covered.

2.   Heat an outdoor grill pan to high temperatures.

3.   Drain the chicken, then pat it dry. Lightly oil the grill grates and cook the chicken for 15 - 20 minutes, frequently flipping, till no longer pink near the bone. Serve with a side salad, cornbread wedges, and your favorite barbecue sauce.

Grilled Wild Duck Breast

(Ready in about 55 minutes | serving 6|Difficulty: Easy)

Per serving: Kcal 297, Fat: 10.7g, Net Carbs: 4.8g, Protein: 43.2g

Ingredients

- Worcestershire sauce ¼ cup
- Olive oil 2 tbsp.
- Hot sauce ½ tsp
- Garlic 2 tbsp., minced
- Black pepper ¼ tsp
- 8 duck breast halves, skinned & boned

Instructions

1. Combine the garlic, Worcestershire sauce, hot sauce, olive oil, and pepper in a mixing bowl. Toss in the duck breasts and coat well. Cover and marinate for at least 30 min to overnight in the refrigerator.

2. Preheat the grill to medium-high.

3. Grill the duck until it's done to your liking, roughly five min per side, based on the size of a breast and the grill temperature.

Delicious Grilled Turkey Burgers

(Ready in about 20 minutes | serving 4|Difficulty: Easy)

Per serving: Kcal 597, Fat: 21.3g, Net Carbs: 45.3g, Protein: 44.4g

Ingredients

- Ground turkey 1 lb.
- Red onion 2 tbsp. Chopped
- Sour cream 2 tbsp.
- Dijon mustard 1 tbsp.
- Montreal steak seasoning 1 tsp
- Olive oil 1 tbsp., or to taste
- To taste, salt
- Swiss cheese 4 slices
- 4 hamburger buns, Hawaiian-style

Instructions

1. Preheat an outdoor grill to medium-high heat and brush the grate liberally with oil.

2. In a mixing bowl, combine the turkey, sour cream, red onion, mustard, and steak seasoning. Make four 3/4-inch thick patties. Season with salt and drizzle with olive oil on both sides.

3. Cook until cooked through on a preheated grill, about Five minutes per side, then top with Swiss cheese shortly before removing from grill. At least 165 degrees F should be read on an instant-read thermometer placed into the center of burgers.

Grilled Turkey Cuban Sandwiches

(Ready in about 2 hours 15 minutes | serving 6|Difficulty: Moderate)

Per serving: Kcal 1066, Fat: 34.4g, Net Carbs: 95.1g, Protein: 91.6g

Ingredients

- cooking spray, Non-stick
- 1 Turkey breast roast (3 lbs.), boneless & thawed
- Garlic 2 cloves, peeled & sliced
- Canola oil 1 tbsp.
- Cumin 1 tbsp. Ground
- Salt 2 tsp
- Black pepper 1 tsp
- 15 inch long loaves Cuban 2, Italian bread
- Honey mustard ¼ cup
- Smoked ham ½ lb.
- Swiss cheese ½ lb.
- 12 slices of dill pickle, sandwich-style

Instructions

1.   Using cooking spray, spray the cold grate of an outdoor gas grill. Make sure the grill is set to medium-low indirect heat.

2.   Take the turkey out of the package. Paper towels can be used to absorb moisture. Refrigerate for 3 days the gravy packet or discard. To make it easier to remove the roast after cooking, lift the string netting and change its position on the roast. Cut slits across the whole surface of the turkey, at least 1-inch apart. Each slit should have 1 garlic slice. Brush the turkey with oil.

3.   Salt, cumin, and pepper should be combined in a bowl. Over the turkey, sprinkle it.

4.   Place the turkey on top of the drip pan on the grill grate. Cover the grill. 1 1/4 - 1 3/4 hours on the grill, or until a meat thermometer inserted into the center of the roast reads 170°F. Take the grill off the heat. Allow 10 minutes for the mixture to cool.

5.   String netting should be removed. Make six 1/8-inch-thick slices from half of the turkey. Unsliced turkey can be kept in the refrigerator for later use.

6.   Make a half-lengthwise cut in each loaf of bread. Cut each one into three pieces after that (for 6 sandwiches). 2 teaspoons mustard, spread on the bottom half of each section. Sliced turkey, cheese, ham, and pickles should be placed on top. Bread loaves tops should be used to cover the tops of the loaves. To flatten the sandwiches, use your hands. Wrap aluminum foil around each item tightly.

7.   Place the sandwiches on the grill grate, wrapped in aluminum foil. A hefty iron skillet or a brick should be placed on top of each one. Grill each side for 3 to 5 minutes, or until thoroughly heated.

8.   Wrapped in aluminum foil, serve sandwiches warm.

Grilled Turkey Asparagus Pesto Paninis

(Ready in about 40 minutes | serving 3|Difficulty: Easy)

Per serving: Kcal 961, Fat: 72.7g, Net Carbs: 37.2g, Protein: 43.1g

Ingredients

For Pesto

- 2 cups basil, chopped & fresh
- Parmesan cheese, ½ cup grated
- ¼ cup olive oil, extra-virgin
- Garlic 2 cloves
- To taste, salt & black pepper
- Pine nuts ¼ cup

For Panini

- Trimmed asparagus spears, 8 fresh
- Butter 2 tbsp., softened
- Oatmeal bread 4 slices, soft
- Provolone cheese 4 slices
- Turkey meat ¼ lb. Sliced

Instructions

1. In a food processor or blender, combine basil, olive oil, Parmesan cheese, garlic, pepper, and salt till smooth, scraping down sides as necessary. Pulse in pine nuts until they are finely chopped but still visible.
2. Preheat the grill over medium-low heat and brush the grate gently with oil.
3. Cook 5 to 10 minutes on a hot grill, directly on the grate, until asparagus is tender.
4. Spread 1 1/2 tsp butter on one side of each slice of bread on the other side of each bread piece, place the required amount of pesto. On the pesto side of two bread pieces, place provolone cheese & turkey; place the second bread piece, side down of pesto.
5. Put sandwiches on the grill & cook for 6 minutes per side, or till cheese is melted and golden brown. Remove the sandwiches from the grill and cut them in half.

Grilled Turkey Legs

(Ready in about 1 hour 15 minutes | serving 4|Difficulty: Easy)
Per serving: Kcal 496, Fat: 9.6g, Net Carbs: 53g, Protein: 49.4g

Ingredients

- Carbonated beverage, lemon-lime flavored, 1 bottle
- Sugar 2 tbsp.
- Hot sauce 2 tbsp.
- Red pepper flakes 1 tbsp., crushed
- Black pepper 1 tbsp.
- Sweet onion 1 large, sliced
- Turkey legs 4
- Honey 2 tbsp.
- Steak seasoning 1 tbsp.

Instructions

1. Preheat an outdoor grill to high heat and brush the grate gently with oil.
2. Combine the pepper, lemon-lime (carbonated beverage), hot sauce, sugar, red pepper, and onion in a big pot. Bring the mixture to a boil, then add the turkey legs. Cook for 30 to 45 minutes, or until the turkey's internal temperature reaches 180 degrees F.
3. Remove the onion slices from the mixture and place them on the grill that has been preheated. Arrange the turkey legs on top of the onions. Sprinkle with steak seasoning and a drizzle of honey. Cook for 20 minutes, flipping once, or until the turkey legs have developed a crisp browned crust.

Turkey Kabobs

(Ready in about 2 hours 30 minutes | serving 4|Difficulty: Moderate)
Per serving: Kcal 480, Fat: 35.3g, Net Carbs: 17.2g, Protein: 26.5g

Ingredients

- Turkey cutlets 1 lb., cut into chunks
- 1 package mushrooms, 16 ounces
- Zucchinis 2 small, sliced
- 1 bottle salad dressing, Italian-style 16 ounces
- Bamboo skewers 12, soaked in water for 15 minutes

Instructions

1. In a dish, combine the mushrooms, turkey, and zucchini. Combine the mixture with the Italian dressing and toss to coat. Cover dish with plastic wrap and marinate for two hours overnight in the refrigerator.
2. Preheat an outdoor grill to medium-high heat and brush the grate liberally with oil.
3. Using skewers, mushrooms, thread turkey, and zucchini slices until all of the items are used. The excess marinade should be discarded.
4. Cook the skewers on the prepared grill, regularly flipping, for about 15 minutes, or until nicely browned on both sides as well as the meat is no longer pink in the center.

Baja-style Rosemary Chicken Skewers

(Ready in about 50 minutes | serving 4|Difficulty: Easy)

Per serving: Kcal 327, Fat: 21.9g, Net Carbs: 1.7g, Protein: 29.6g

Ingredients

- White onion 1/2 small, finely chopped
- Minced garlic 3 cloves
- Chiles de arbol 2 dried
- Minced rosemary 1 tsp
- Mexican oregano 1 tsp, crumbled
- 1/4 cup lemon juice
- 1/4 cup olive oil (extra-virgin)
- 2 lbs. Chicken thighs, boneless & skinless
- Kosher salt & pepper
- 8 rosemary sprigs 12 inch
- For serving, lime wedges

Instructions

1. Combine the onion, chiles, garlic, rosemary, lemon juice, oregano, and olive oil in a large mixing bowl. Add the chicken to the bowl after seasoning it with salt and pepper. Mix thoroughly, cover, and set aside for 30 minutes to marinade.

2. Preheat the grill. Remove the pieces of chicken from the marinade and thread them onto rosemary skewers; remove the marinade. Grill the chicken on moderate heat, rotating frequently and basting with the remaining marinade, for 15 to 20 minutes, till golden and cooked through. Serve with lemon wedges on the side.

PART 3: BEEF RECIPES

Perfect Grilled Steak

(Ready in about 90 minutes | serving 2-3|Difficulty: Easy)

Per serving: Kcal 327, Fat: 21.9g, Net Carbs: 1.7g, Protein: 29.6g

Ingredients

- 2 large ribeye steaks (about 2 pounds), 1.7-2.2 inches thick
- ground black pepper to taste
- salt to taste

Instructions

1.   Season steaks with salt. Let it rest on a plate for at least 40 minutes (or up to 4 days). If you'd like a seasoning longer than 40 minutes, transfer to a wire rack set in a rimmed baking sheet and place uncovered in refrigerator, until ready to cook.

2.   Light the charcoal and when all charcoal is lit and covered with gray ash, move coals on one side of charcoal grate. Place the cooking to cover the grill, and preheat for 5 minutes. Clean the grilling grate and oil it.

3.   Complete the steak seasoning with pepper and place on cooler side of grill. Cover and cook, with all vents open, flipping and checking temperature every few minutes with an instant-read thermometer. When the steaks register 105°F (41°C) for medium-rare or 115°F (46°C) for medium, they're ready, 10 to 15 minutes total.

4.   Move steaks to the hottest side of grill and cook, flipping frequently, until a deep char has appeared and internal temperature registers 125°F (52°C) for medium-rare or 135°F (57°C) for medium, about 2 minutes total.

5.   Place steaks to a cutting board and let it rest for at least 5 to 10 minutes. Slice and serve immediately.

Slow-Smoked Chuck Perfection

(Ready in about 12 hours | serving 9|Difficulty: Difficult)

Per serving: Kcal 327, Fat: 21.9g, Net Carbs: 1.7g, Protein: 29.6g

Ingredients

- 1 piece beef chuck roll (4/5 pound)
- 1/4 cup salt

- 2 ounces ground black peppercorns

For Serving:

- white bread
- dill pickles

- yellow onion, sliced

Instructions

1.   In a small bowl, combine salt and pepper. Rub the mixture over the surface of the chuck roll. Tie 2 to 3 pieces of twine around the chuck roll circumference at 1- to 1 1/2-inch intervals.

2.   Light the charcoal and once lit and covered with gray ash, arrange coals on one side. Set cooking grate in place, and preheat for 5 minutes. If you're using a gas grill, set half the burners to medium-high heat, cover, and preheat for 10 minutes. Clean and oil the grill.

3.   Use the cooler side of grill to start cooking your roll, but add 4 hardwood chunks to the hotter side. (If you're using a gas grill, wrap wood chunks loosely in aluminum foil before carefully placing over the hotter side). Cover and allow beef to smoke. Make sure to maintain a temperature between 275 and 300°F (135 and 149°C) adjusting vents and adding coals a few at a time or adjusting the knobs on a gas grill as needed. Add 2 to 3 wood chunks twice during cooking. When a deep, dark bark has formed and the internal temperature reaches between 150 and 165°F (66 and 74°C), the smoking is finished (about 4 hours).

4.   Remove the beef and wrap tightly in a double layer of heavy-duty aluminum foil. Pu it back to the cooler side of the grill and keep adding coals or adjusting knobs to sustain internal grill temperature between 225 and 250°F (107 and 121°C). As an alternative, you can relocate the foil-wrapped chuck to a wire rack set in a rimmed baking sheet and finish the cooking in a preheated 225°F (107°C) oven indoors. (Downside: your house will have a stong smoke smell for a while).

5.   Cook 5 to 5 1/2 hours longer, when the meat is almost completely tender and a fork inserted and twisted will show little resistance. Remove the foil and return the meat to the grill or oven, and continue cooking for about 30 minutes or until a crisp bark forms.

6.   Remove from heat, transfer to a cutting board, cover with foil, and let it cool until internal temperature drops to between 140 and 165°F (60 and 74°C) before serving.

7.   When it's time to serve, slice in half running knife in between the two massive muscle groups to part them. Get rid of twine and set the two halves cut side down on the cutting board.

8.   Using a sharp knife, cut meat thinly against the grain and serve with pickles, sliced onion, and white bread. Slice only what you are serving; the uneaten leftover can be wrapped in foil and refrigerated for up to 1 week. Reheat the remaining chuck for about 1 hour in a 275°F (135°C) oven directly in the foil.

(Ready in about 90 minutes | serving 4|Difficulty: Easy)

Per serving: Kcal 327, Fat: 21.9g, Net Carbs: 1.7g, Protein: 29.6g

Ingredients

- 2 pounds skirt steak (fat trimmed ready)
- 1/4 cup orange juice
- 2 tablespoons juice from 2 limes, plus 1 extra lime for serving
- 1 teaspoon ground cumin
- 2/3 cup olive oil
- 4 medium cloves garlic, minced
- 1/4 cup fresh cilantro leaves and fine stems, chopped
- freshly ground black pepper and Kosher salt

Instructions

1. Pour lime and orange juices, cumin, 1 teaspoon salt, 1/3 cup olive oil, garlic, and 1/2 teaspoon pepper in a resealable bag, and insert the skirt steak in it. Seal, squish and massage to marinate. Let it rest in the refrigerator at least 1 hour and up to overnight.

2. When ready to cook, remove from marinade and pat dry with paper towels. Pour the marinade into a small saucepan and simmer over medium heat until it's reduced by half.

3. Light the charcoal and once lit and covered with gray ash, arrange coals on one side. As always, set the cooking grate in place, and preheat for 5 minutes. If you're using a gas grill, set half the burners to medium-high heat, cover, and preheat for 10 minutes. Clean and oil the grill.

4. Place the skirt steak on the hot side of the grill and cook, flipping every 30 seconds, until brown-charred. And when an instant-read thermometer inserted into their center indicates 115°F to 120°F for medium-rare or 125°F to 130°F for medium, it's time to lay your steak to a large plate, cover in foil, and let it rest for 10 minutes.

5. Slice against the muscle fibers, sprinkle with pan sauce and cilantro. Serve with extra lime wedges.

Carne Asada Juicy Dish

(Ready in about 4 hours | serving 6|Difficulty: Easy)

Per serving: Kcal 327, Fat: 21.9g, Net Carbs: 1.7g, Protein: 29.6g

Ingredients

- 2 pounds skirt steak (2 to 3 whole skirt steaks), sliced into 5- to 6-inch lengths
- 3 whole dried guajillo chiles
- 3 whole dried ancho chiles
- 3/4 cup fresh juice from 2 to 3 oranges
- 2 whole chipotle peppers
- 2 tablespoons extra-virgin olive oil
- 2 tablespoons fresh juice from 2 to 3 limes
- 2 tablespoons Asian fish sauce
- 2 tablespoons soy sauce
- 1 small bunch cilantro
- 1 teaspoon whole coriander seed, toasted
- 1 tablespoon whole cumin seed, toasted
- 6 medium cloves garlic
- 2 tablespoons dark brown sugar
- Kosher salt
- Warm corn or flour tortillas, diced onion, fresh cilantro, lime wedges, and avocado for serving

Instructions

1. Microwave the dried ancho and guajillo chiles 10 to 20 seconds on a microwave-safe plate. Put them in a blender with orange juice, chipotle peppers, lime juice, soy sauce, olive oil, fish sauce, cumin seed, coriander seed, garlic, cilantro, and brown sugar. Blend for about 1 minute, until you have a smooth sauce. Add salt to taste. Pour half of the salsa into a large bowl. The other half into a sealed container, and set aside in the refrigerator.

2. Let's make the salsa in the bowl slightly saltier than is comfortable to taste by adding an extra 2 teaspoons of salt. Place 1 steak into a bowl, turn and massage to coat. Transfer to a gallon-sized zipper-lock bag (fold the top over to prevent excess sauce and meat juices from contaminating the seal). Repeat the procedure with the remaining steak, and add them to the same bag. Drain all excess marinade over the steaks, before squeezing all air out of the bag, then seal. Place in refrigerator for at least 3 hours (and up to overnight).

3. When it's time to cook, remove the extra salsa from the fridge and leave it uncool until the grill is ready. Light the charcoal and once lit and covered with gray ash, arrange coals on one side. As always, set the cooking grate in place, and preheat for 5 minutes. If you're using a gas grill, set half the burners to medium-high heat, cover, and preheat for 10 minutes. Clean and oil the grill.

4. Get the steaks out of the bags and wipe off sauce excess. Place it directly over the grill's hot side. If you're using a gas grill, cover; if using a charcoal grill instead, leave exposed.

5. Cook, and turn every 30 seconds for better inside cooking, until the outside is well charred and your instant-read thermometer reads 110°F in the steak center (5 to 10 minutes total).

6. Allow to rest for 5 minutes on a cutting board, then slice thinly against the grain and serve immediately, arranging the side ingredients around. Enjoy!

Preparation Time:10 Minutes

Cooking Time:10 Minutes

Servings:4

Ingredients:

- 4 ribeye steaks, fat trimmed, 1-1⁄2-inch thick slices
- 2 teaspoons ground black pepper
- 2 teaspoons salt

For the Seasoning:

- 2 teaspoons smoked paprika
- 2 tablespoon erythritol sweetener
- 1 teaspoon red flavored
- 1 teaspoon turmeric powder
- 4 tablespoons steak seasoning

Directions:

1. Season the steak with salt and black pepper, massage the meat for 3-5 minutes.
2. Prepare the grill by lighting the charcoals, until it's covered by ash. Move them on one side, put the cooking grate in place, cover, and allow to preheat for five minutes. Oil it.
3. Place 1 steak onto cooler side of the cooking grate and sear it for 3 minutes. Flip it and cook for 3 minutes.
4. Transfer it to the hotter side of the grate, close the lid, and flip occasionally for additional 3 minutes, or until the thermometer registers 140°F for medium-rare, or 155°F for a medium-cooked steak. Repeat with the remaining steaks.
5. Remove the steaks from the grill, cover them with foil and let them cool off for five minutes.
6. Slice against the grain and serve!

Nutrition:

629 Cal; 41 g Fats; 58 g Protein; 8 g Net Carb; 1 g Fiber

The Sweet-love Burger

Preparation Time:25 Minutes

Cooking Time:1 Hour and 20 Minutes

Servings:6

Ingredients:

For the Maple Bacon:
- 12 slices bacon
- ¼ cup pure maple syrup
- 1/3 cup light brown sugar, packed

For the Candied Jalapenos:
- 2 large jalapeno peppers, sliced into rounds
- 1/3 cup granulated sugar
- ¼ cup distilled white vinegar

For the Burgers:
- 12 ounces ground beef chuck
- 6 ounces ground beef sirloin
- 6 slices mozzarella cheese
- 6 slices provolone cheese
- 6 slices Swiss cheese
- 6 sesame brioche buns, split
- 6 ounces ground beef brisket
- 1/3 cup seltzer
- Unsalted butter, for spreading
- A pinch of Cajun seasoning
- Vegetable oil, for the grill
- Freshly ground pepper & kosher salt to taste
- Butter lettuce, sliced tomatoes, and sliced avocado, for topping

Directions:

1.   To prepare the Maple Bacon preheat your oven to 275 F. Place the bacon on a rimmed baking sheet & bake for 30 minutes; brush with some maple syrup and sprinkle with brown sugar. Bake until the sugar melts. Extract and allow it to cool.

2.   In a small bowl, mix the jalapenos with vinegar and granulated sugar, then set aside.

3.   To prepare the burgers, go through the preheat procedure and oil the grill. In a large bowl unite beef chuck together with brisket and sirloin, the Cajun seasoning, seltzer & a pinch each of salt and pepper. Combine the mixture with your hand and make six patties, approximately ½" thick.

4.   Grill the burgers for 3 ½ minutes; flip and top each with a slice of provolone, Swiss cheese, and mozzarella. Cover and cook for 2 ½ minutes more.

5.   While they cook, butter the cut sides of the buns and grill them for one minute, on the cooler side of the grate.

6.   Garnish with candied jalapenos, avocado, maple bacon, lettuce, and tomato.

Nutrition:

887 calories 59g total fats 43g protein

Southern Style Burger

Preparation Time:15 Minutes
Cooking Time:30 Minutes
Servings:4

Ingredients:
- 2 pounds ground bison or beef
- 1 small onion, minced
- 4 garlic cloves, minced
- 1 tablespoon Texas Pete or Tabasco
- 1 large green tomato, cut into 8 slices
- BBQ Sauce with Honey and Molasses
- 1 large egg, beaten
- 8 ounces container pimento cheese spread
- 1/4 cup corn meal, seasoned with salt and pepper
- Pickled okra for condiments
- 8 Hearty Buns
- Cooking spray

Directions:
1.   Preheat your oven to 350 degrees. Pour a small amount of water in a shallow bowl, mix in the egg and season with salt and pepper to taste. Set the corn meal out onto a medium-sized plate close by.
2.   Soak the tomato slices into the egg mixture and right away press them into the corn meal; make sure that the outside is completely coated.
3.   Spray the nonstick cooking spray on the baking sheet and place the slices on it. Diffuse also the tops of tomatoes with some cooking spray. Bake until golden brown, for 12 to 15 minutes, turning once during the baking process.
4.   In a large-sized mixing bowl, combine the ground beef together with onions, garlic and tabasco. Season the meat and combine thoroughly. Create 8 even-sized patties from this mixture. Use the BBQ Sauce to baste the patties and grill until you get your desired doneness.
5.   Use a cookie scoop to place a portion of pimento cheese spread on top of burgers, about one minute before you remove the patties from the grill. Press the cheese down using a large spatula for even melting.
6.   Arrange one "fried" green tomato over each bun, add a burger on top, and garnish with condiments of your liking.

Nutrition:
893 calories 58g total fats 40g protein

Preparation Time:15 Minutes
Cooking Time:15 Minutes
Servings:4

Ingredients:
- 1 ½ pounds ground beef
- 1 tablespoon butter

Tex-Mex seasoning:
- 2 tablespoons paprika
- 2 teaspoons ground cumin
- ½ teaspoon cayenne pepper
- 1 teaspoon black pepper
- 4 slices Applewood-smoked bacon, cooked and

Pico de Gallo:
- 1-2 Roma tomatoes, deseeded and diced thin
- 1-2 teaspoons fresh cilantro, finely chopped
- ½-1 tablespoon thinly diced red onion
- 1-2 teaspoons fresh lime juice
- 1-2 teaspoons jalapeños pepper, thinly diced

For serving (optional)
- Guacamole, and sour cream

- 8 (6-inch) flour tortillas

- crumbled
- 1 tablespoon dried oregano Toppings
- 8 slices pepper jack cheese
- 1 teaspoon salt or to taste
- ½ cup shredded iceberg lettuce

- ½ cup ranch dressing such as Hidden Valley
- ½ cup sour cream
- 1 teaspoon Tex-Mex seasoning
- ¼ cup mild salsa
- Salt and pepper to taste

Directions:
1.   Combine the Tex-Mex seasoning ingredients in a mixing bowl, and stir to make sure they are well combined.
2.   Mix all the ingredients in a second bowl to prepare the Pico de Gallo. Set aside and refrigerate until you need to use it.
3.   Sprinkle 2 tablespoons of the Tex-Mex seasoning onto the ground beef and blend it in. Create 4 large ¼-inch thick burger patties and cook them on the grill. Be careful not to overcook the beef, they should reach 380°F.
4.   Butter each of the tortillas on one side. Set one butter side down in a pre-heated skillet. Top with one slice of cheese, some shredded lettuce, bacon, Pico de Gallo, and top with a cooked burger. Add a drizzle of the Tex-Mex ranch dressing, bacon, Pico the Gallo, and another slice of cheese. Finish by topping with another tortilla, butter side up. Cook until the tortilla is golden, for about 1 minute.
5.   Carefully flip the tortilla and cook until you see the cheese melting. You can also use a sandwich press if you prefer.
6.   Cut the tortillas in halves and serve with a side of guacamole, sour cream, and Tex-Mex ranch dressing. Enjoy!

Nutrition:
725 calories 12g fats 34g protein

Preparation Time:20 Minutes

Cooking Time:10 Minutes

Servings:2

Ingredients:

- 2 sirloin steaks, (6-ounce)
- 2 teaspoons blackened steak seasoning
- 2 tablespoons unsalted butter
- 1/2 cup sliced green peppers
- 1/2 cup sliced red peppers
- 2 cloves garlic, minced
- 1 cup yellow onion, sliced
- 2 slices Monterey jack cheese
- 2 slices cheddar cheese
- Salt and Pepper, to taste
- Vegetable medley or garlic mashed potatoes, for side

Directions:

1. Season both side of the sirloin steak with blackened seasoning and let it rest for 15 minutes.
2. Prepare the grill by lighting the charcoals, until it's covered by ash. Move them on one side, put the cooking grate in place, cover, and allow to preheat for five minutes. Oil it.
3. Cook the steak directly over heat for 6 minutes per side, or until it reaches an internal temperature of 140°F for a medium-rare or 155°F for a medium-cooked steak.
4. Using a skillet, melt the butter and cook the onion, peppers, and garlic. Add salt and pepper to taste.
5. One minute before the steak has reached your desired doneness, top it with a slice of each cheese. You'll see the cheese melting.
6. Let it rest for 1 minute, then pour over the onion & peppers mix.
7. Serve the steaks with the garlic mashed potatoes or the mixed vegetables side.

Nutrition:

679 calories 12g fats 32g protein

Preparation Time:10 Minutes

Cooking Time:20 Minutes

Servings:4

Ingredients:

Steak ingredients

- 4 1-inch thick New York strip steaks
- 5 tablespoons soy sauce
- 1 quart beef stock
- 1/4 cup apple cider vinegar
- 6 tablespoons Worcestershire sauce
- 4 teaspoons meat tenderizer
- 2 tablespoons smoked paprika

- 1 1/2 tablespoons minced garlic
- 1 1/2 tablespoons chili powder
- 1 1/2 tablespoons black pepper
- 2 teaspoons cayenne pepper
- 2 teaspoons onion salt
- 1 teaspoon dried oregano

Other ingredients

- 1 1/2 cups sliced mushrooms
- 1 onion, sliced
- 1 tablespoon butter

- 4 large potatoes, cut into 1-inch cubes
- 2 garlic cloves, minced
- Oil for deep frying

Directions:

1.   Get yourself a large resealable bag or container with a lid, combine all the ingredients and mix to make sure they form a consistent marinade. Insert the steak too, cover with the mix, massage it and refrigerate for 8 hours up to overnight, turning the bag a couple of times.

2.   Heat the frying oil in a saucepot until it reaches 350F. If you have a deep fryer, turn it on so the oil is ready.

3.   Prepare the grill by lighting the charcoals, until it's covered by ash. Move them on one side, put the cooking grate in place, cover, and allow to preheat for five minutes. Oil it.

4.   Cook the steaks to your preference, about 4 minutes per side, or until it reaches 135°F for medium-rare or 145°F for medium. Transfer to a plate and tent with foil.

5.   While steaks are cooking, melt the butter in a skillet over medium heat. Add onions and sauté for 2 minutes. Add the mushrooms and continue cooking until they get golden, for about 4 minutes.

6.   At the same time, fry the potatoes for about 6-8 minutes, until, golden brown. Remove them from oil and place them in paper towel to absorb excess oil. Add salt, and if desired, paprika.

7.   Arrange mushrooms and onions next to the steak and add the potatoes. Enjoy!

Nutrition:

641 calories 9g fats 34g protein

Peppercorn Cheese Steak

Preparation Time:10 Minutes
Cooking Time:8 to 10 Minutes
Servings:4

Ingredients:

- 4 sirloin steaks (7-ounce)
- ½ cup Asiago cheese, shredded
- 1 tablespoon cracked black peppercorns
- 4 red potatoes, roasted, for serving
- Salt to taste
- 1-pound seasonal vegetables, steamed

Directions:

1.   Prepare the grill by lighting the charcoals, until it's covered by ash. Move them on one side, put the cooking grate in place, cover, and allow to preheat for five minutes.
2.   Drizzle salt and peppercorns to season the steak and let it rest for 15 minutes.
3.   Grill the steaks to your desired doneness, 3–4 minutes on each side, flipping every minute until the temperature reaches 135°F for medium-rare or 145°F for medium.
4.   When the temperature is about to be reached, sprinkle steak with 2 tablespoon of Asiago cheese, close the lid and wait 1 minute for the cheese to melt.
5.   Serve with a side of preferred vegetables and a roasted potato.

Nutrition:
684 calories 9g fats 31g protein

Onion & Mushroom Burger

Preparation Time:10 Minutes
Cooking Time:20 Minutes
Servings:4

Ingredients:

- 1 lb. ground hamburger
- ½ onion caramelized
- 2 c. mushrooms, sliced
- 1 tbsp. butter
- 4 slices Swiss cheese
- Lettuce
- Onion powder to taste
- Garlic salt to taste
- Seasoned salt to taste

Directions:

1.   Prepare the grill by lighting the charcoals, until it's covered by ash, and allow to preheat for five minutes, until it reaches medium heat.
2.   Mold 8 even balls out of the hamburgers, adding a pinch of onion powder to each ball. Flat and season both sides of each with both salts.
3.   Grill until the meat reaches 380°F, or up to your desired doneness.
4.   In the meanwhile caramelize the onions and sauté the mushrooms with butter until tender.
5.   When the burgers are ready, remove them from the heat and let them cool as you top them with the onions & mushrooms. Arrange lettuce and cheese as sides.

Nutrition:
891 calories 58.9g total fats 37.9g protein

Big Chief Burger

Preparation Time:

15 Minutes

Cooking Time:

25 Minutes

Servings:

3

Ingredients:

- 1-pound ground beef
- 6 bacon slices, cooked until crisp
- 3 fried eggs
- 3 Cheddar cheese slices
- Verde green sauce or canned green chilis
- Worcestershire sauce
- Pico de Gallo
- 3 burger buns
- Salt and Pepper to taste

Directions:

1. Prepare the grill by lighting the charcoals, until it's covered by ash, and allow to preheat for five minutes, until it reaches high heat.

2. Season the ground beef with salt and pepper, and splashes of Worcestershire sauce. Form 3 patties with the mixture and cook until they reach 380°F, or up to your desired level of doneness.

3. During the last minute of cooking, top each burger with a cheese slice so that it starts to get soft and melt.

4. Remove from heat and top with 1 fried egg, 2 slices of bacon, a generous scoop of Pico de Gallo, and 1 tablespoon of Verde sauce. Serve immediately and enjoy!

Nutrition:

889 calories 60g total fats 40g protein

Spicy Avocado Beef Burger

Preparation Time:20 Minutes

Cooking Time:20 Minutes

Servings:4

Ingredients:

- 1-pound ground beef
- 2 avocados
- 8 sliced crispy cooked bacon
- 1 teaspoon Worcestershire sauce
- 8 Tomato slices
- 4 Onion Slices
- 4 slices of American cheese
- 1/4 teaspoon dried thyme
- 1 teaspoon Tabasco sauce
- Fresh Lettuce
- Mayonnaise
- 4 sesame burger buns
- Salt and pepper to taste

Directions:

1.   Season the ground beef with Worcestershire sauce, salt, tabasco, thyme, and pepper, by carefully tossing the ingredients with a fork until well combined. Create 4 palm-sized beef patties from the compound.

2.   Prepare the grill by lighting the charcoals, until it's covered by ash, and allow to preheat for five minutes, until it reaches medium heat.

3.   When the grill is ready, grill the beef patties for about 4 minutes per side until they reach 380°F, or up to your desired level of doneness.

4.   While they're cooking, mash the avocado and season with 1 pinch of salt and pepper.

5.   Spread a thin layer of mayonnaise on the bottom half of the bun and lay lettuce, 1 onion slice, and 1 tomato slice over it. Add the hot beef patty and top it with cheese. Add 2 slices of crispy bacon over it.

6.   Spread the avocado sauce over the cut part of the top bun, before topping it all. Serve immediately and enjoy!

Nutrition:

907 calories 61g total fats 40g protein

Soft Cheese & Steak Bagel Sandwich

Preparation Time: 32 minutes Cooking Time: 9 minutes Serving: 2

Ingredients

- 1 beef cube steak
- 1 tsp. onion
- 2 eggs
- 2 slices American cheese
- 2 tbsp. Worcestershire sauce
- 2 tbsp. butter
- 1 1/2 tsp. garlic salt
- 2 split bagels
- Nonstick cooking spray

Directions:

1. Mix the Worcestershire sauce, garlic salt, and onion in a resealable bag. When well combined insert the steak and massage, and leave it marinade, for at least 15 minutes.

2. Prepare the grill by lighting the charcoals, until it's covered by ash, and allow to preheat for five minutes, until it reaches medium heat.

3. When ready, cook the steak for 6 minutes, flipping it midway, until it reaches 360°F, or until it gets to your desired doneness.

4. In the meantime, butter the insides of the bagel and toast it for 2 minutes on the cooler side of the grill.

5. Beat the eggs in a small bowl. Spray a skillet and cook the eggs. When ready, fold in half like an omelet and slice into 4 equal pieces.

6. Place the cooked steak on the bottom half of the bagel, top it with egg and cheese, and close it with the remaining half of the bagel.

Nutrition

270 Calories 22g Fat 20g Protein

Tacos Steak

Preparation Time: 40 min Cooking Time: 15 minutes Servings: 6

Ingredients:
- 1.5 lb. Beef flank steak
- 6 Whole wheat tortillas (8-inches)
- 2 Large tomatoes
- 1 Jalapeno pepper
- 1 large slice Onion
- 0.25 cup Lime juice
- 0.5 cup Red onion
- 3 tablespoon Fresh cilantro
- 0.75 teaspoon Salt
- 2 teaspoon Ground cumin
- 1 teaspoon Canola oil
- Optional: sliced avocado, lime wedges

Directions:

1.   Chop and deseed the jalapeno and tomatoes. Dice the onion and chop cilantro.

2.   For the salsa combine the lime juice, onion, cilantro, tomatoes and jalapeno. Stir in one teaspoon of cumin and add 1/4 teaspoon of salt. Set aside.

3.   Season the steak with the rest of the salt and cumin, and let it rest for 15 minutes.

4.   Prepare the grill and cook using medium temperature with the lid on for 6-8 minutes, or until the steak is of your desired doneness (the instant-read thermometer, will be about 135°F for a medium-rare). Let it rest and cool down for five minutes before slicing.

5.   Warm the Canola oil in a skillet at med-high temperature and sauté the onion until it is crisp but tender.

6.   Slice the steak in thin slices across the grain and serve on tortillas with onion and salsa. Serve with lime wedges and avocado.

Nutrition:

Calories: 329 Protein: 27 grams Fat: 12 grams Sat. Fats: 4 grams Carbohydrates: 29 grams Sugars: 3 grams Fiber: 5 grams

Preparation Time: 10 minutes Cooking Time: 20 minutes Servings: 6

Ingredients:

- 18 ounces rib eye or sirloin steak, cut into 2–3-inch medallions
- 4 cups baby spinach
- 1-pound fettuccine
- 1⁄2 cup gorgonzola cheese, crumbled
- 1⁄2 cup sun-dried tomatoes, chopped
- Balsamic glaze (or aged balsamic)

Alfredo sauce

- 3 tablespoons all-purpose flour
- 3 tablespoons butter
- 1⁄2 cup pecorino romano cheese, grated
- 2 cups heavy cream

Directions:

1. Prepare the grill by lighting the charcoals, until it's covered by ash, and allow to preheat for five minutes, until it reaches medium heat.

2. In the meanwhile make the alfredo sauce by melting the butter in a saucepan over medium heat. Add the flour, slowly and whisking frequently. Pour in the heavy cream and the grated cheese, and continue to whisk until thickened yet smooth.

3. Cook fettuccine according to directions on the package. Drain and set aside.

4. Grill the meat to preference. If you're cooking the sirloin steak check for an internal temperature of 135°F for medium-rare and 145°F for medium. If you're cooking the rib eye grill 8 minutes per side or to 140°F for med-rare or 10 minutes per side or to 155°F for medium.

5. Heat the alfredo sauce in a pot on low. Add the pasta and spinach and continue to stir until the spinach wilts, then remove from heat.

6. Top the cooked meat with sun-dried tomatoes, and gorgonzola cheese. Drizzle with balsamic glaze.

7. Place the meat at the center of a plate and arrange the pasta around it. Serve and Enjoy!

Nutrition:

497 calories 7.9g carbohydrates 32g protein

Herb Crusted Royal Tenderloin

Preparation Time: 50 minutes Cooking Time: 40 minutes Servings: 6

Ingredients:

- 3.5 lb tenderloin, trimmed
- 2 tablespoon thyme, minced
- 2 tablespoon rosemary, minced
- 4 cloves garlic, minced
- 1/3 cup extra virgin olive oil

Directions:

1. Let the beef tenderloin rest at room temperature for about 15 mins before grilling.
2. Tie the beef tenderloin off using kitchen twine in 1 inch intervals.
3. Prepare the grill by lighting the charcoals, until it's covered by ash. Move them on one side, put the cooking grate in place, cover, and allow to preheat for five minutes.
4. Season the tenderloin all around with salt and pepper.
5. Blend the garlic, herbs, and olive oil in a tiny bowl (use a blender for a finer result) and spread the herb mixture all over the beef tenderloin on all sides.
6. Move the beef tenderloin to the hotter side of the grill and sear on all sides 10 minutes in total.
7. Transfer the tenderloin to the cooler side, cover, and cook for about 30 mins, or until the temperature reaches 130°F for medium rare, .
8. Take the sirloin off the heat and move it to a tray. Let the meat rest for 20 mins under some foil. Cut the strings and slice. Enjoy!

Nutrition:

628 calories 1g carbohydrates 37g protein

PART 4: LAMB RECIPES

Grilled Leg of Lamb Steaks

(Ready in about 50 minutes | serving 4|Difficulty: Easy)

Per serving: Kcal 327, Fat: 21.9g, Net Carbs: 1.7g, Protein: 29.6g

Ingredients

- 4 lamb steaks, bone-in
- Olive oil ¼ cup
- Garlic 4 cloves, minced
- Chopped rosemary 1 tbsp., fresh
- To taste, salt & black pepper

Instructions

1. In a shallow dish, put lamb steaks in a single layer. Olive oil, rosemary, garlic, salt, and pepper are drizzled over the top. To cover both sides of the steaks, flip them. Allow 30 minutes for the steaks to absorb the seasonings.

2. Preheat an outdoor grill to high heat and brush the grate gently with oil. Cook steaks for 5 minutes per side for medium, or till brown on the outside and slightly pink. At least 140 degrees F should be read on an instant-read thermometer placed into the center.

Simple Grilled Lamb Chops

(Ready in about 2 hours 15 minutes | serving 4|Difficulty: Moderate)

Per serving: Kcal 519, Fat: 44.8g, Net Carbs: 2.3g, Protein: 25g

Ingredients

- White vinegar ¼ cup, distilled
- Salt 2 tsp
- Garlic 1 tbsp., minced
- Black pepper ½ tsp
- Onion 1, thinly sliced
- Olive oil 2 tbsp.
- Lamb chops 2 lbs

Instructions

1. In a big resealable bag, combine the onion, vinegar, pepper, salt, garlic, and olive oil till the salt has dissolved. Add the lamb, stir to coat, and marinate for 2 hours in the refrigerator.

2. Preheat the outdoor grill to medium-high.

3. Remove the lamb from the marinade, but don't throw away any onions that have stuck to the meat. Any leftover marinade should be discarded. To keep the exposed ends of bones from burning, wrap them in aluminum foil. Grill until done to your liking, about Three minutes on each side for medium.

Grilled Spicy Lamb Burgers

(Ready in about 25 minutes | serving 4|Difficulty: Easy)

Per serving: Kcal 478, Fat: 22.4g, Net Carbs: 38g, Protein: 29.4g

- Ground lamb 1 lb.
- Mint leaves 2 tbsp., chopped & fresh
- Cilantro 2 tbsp., chopped & fresh
- 2 tbsp. Oregano, chopped & fresh
- Garlic 1 tbsp., chopped
- Sherry 1 tsp
- White wine vinegar 1 tsp
- Molasses 1 tsp
- Cumin 1 tsp, ground
- Allspice ¼ tsp, ground
- Red pepper flakes ½ tsp
- Salt, ½ tsp
- Pita bread 4 rounds
- Black pepper ½ tsp, ground
- Feta cheese 4 ounces, crumbled

Instructions

1. Preheat the grill to medium.

2. Combine the lamb, cilantro, mint, oregano, sherry, garlic, vinegar, and molasses in a large mixing bowl. Mix in the cumin, red pepper flakes, allspice, salt, and black pepper until all are well combined. Shape into four patties.

3. Using a brush, coat the grill grate in oil. Grill for 5 minutes per side, or until burgers are cooked through. Heat each pita pocket on the grill for a few minutes. Serve feta cheese-wrapped burgers in pitas.

Grilled Lamb Loin Chops

(Ready in about 1 hour 20 minutes | serving 6|Difficulty: Easy)

Per serving: Kcal 579, Fat: 43.9g, Net Carbs: 0.7g, Protein: 42.5g

Ingredients

- Herbes de Provence 2 tbsp.
- Olive oil 1 ½ tbsp.
- Garlic 2 cloves, minced
- Lemon juice 2 tsp
- loin chops, 5 ounces
- Salt & black pepper, 1 pinch

Instructions

1. In a small bowl, combine the herbes de Provence, garlic, olive oil, and lemon juice. Put it in the fridge for at least one hour after rubbing the mixture on the lamb chops.

2. Preheat an outdoor grill to medium-high heat and brush the grate liberally with oil.

3. Chops should be seasoned with pepper and salt.

4. Place the chops on the prepared grill and cook for 3 to 4 minutes per side, until browned & medium-rare on the inside. Remove off the grill and set aside for 5 minutes to rest on an aluminum foil-covered dish before serving.

Grilled Lemon and Rosemary Lamb Chops

(Ready in about 4 hours 25 minutes | serving 6|Difficulty: Difficult)

Per serving: Kcal 198, Fat: 13.6g, Net Carbs: 4.5g, Protein: 15.3g

Ingredients

- Plain yogurt ½ cup
- Lemon 1 large, juiced & rind grated
- Chile paste 1 tbsp.
- Garlic 4 cloves, crushed
- Rosemary 2 tbsp., minced & fresh
- Oregano 1 tsp, dried
- Salt & Black pepper
- Cinnamon ¼ tsp ground
- Lamb loin chops, 5 ounces

Instructions

1. In a small bowl, combine yogurt, lemon zest, lemon juice, Chile paste, rosemary, garlic, oregano, black pepper, salt, and cinnamon. Fill a resealable plastic bag halfway with the mixture. Add the lamb chops to the bag, coat them in the marinade, squeeze out excess air, and close it. Refrigerate for 4 hours to marinate.
2. Preheat the grill to medium heat and brush the grate gently with oil.
3. Scrape out any extra marinade from the lamb chops. Remove the marinade that has been used and discard it. Chops should be seasoned with salt and pepper. Place on the hot grill and cook for 3 to 4 minutes, just until browned and medium-rare, mostly on the inside. A thermometer placed into the middle should read 130 degrees F.

Grilled Lamb with Brown Sugar Glaze

(Ready in about 1 hour 25 minutes | serving 4|Difficulty: Easy)

Per serving: Kcal 241, Fat: 13.1g, Net Carbs: 15.8g, Protein: 14.6g

Ingredients

- Brown sugar ¼ cup
- Ginger 2 tsp, ground
- Tarragon 2 tsp, dried
- The ground cinnamon, 1 tsp
- Black pepper 1 tsp, ground
- Garlic powder 1 tsp
- Salt, ½ tsp
- Lamb chops 4

Instructions

1. Combine brown sugar, tarragon, ginger, cinnamon, garlic powder, pepper, and salt in a medium mixing bowl. Season the lamb chops and arrange them on a platter. Put it in the fridge for 1 hour after covering.
2. Preheat the grill to high.
3. Brush the grill grate generously with oil before placing the lamb chops on it. Cook for 5 mins, or until done to your liking.

Grilled Lamb Chops with Pomegranate-Port Reduction

(Ready in about 1 hour 10 minutes | serving 4|Difficulty: Easy)

Per serving: Kcal 396, Fat: 23.4g, Net Carbs: 10.2g, Protein: 25.9g

Ingredients

- Lemon 1, juiced & zested
- 2 tbsp. Oregano, chopped & fresh
- Garlic 2 cloves, minced
- To taste, salt & black pepper
- Lamb chops, 3 ounces
- ½ cup pomegranate juice, fresh & unsweetened
- Port wine 1 cup
- Pomegranate seeds 2 tbsp.

Instructions

1. In a large mixing bowl, combine the lemon juice and zest, oregano, salt, garlic, and black pepper; transfer to a resealable plastic bag. Add the lamb chops to the bag, coat them in the marinade, squeeze out excess air, and seal it. Allow marinating for a while.
2. Preheat an outdoor grill to medium-high heat and brush the grate liberally with oil.
3. In a medium saucepan over high heat, bring the port wine and pomegranate juice to a simmer. Adjust heat to medium-low and continue to simmer for 45 minutes, or until liquid has reduced almost half its original volume. Set aside the pomegranate seeds after stirring them in.⒪⒝⒥
4. Remove the lamb from the marinade and shake off any remaining marinade. Remove the remaining marinade and toss it out. Cook the chops on the hot grill for 4 minutes per side for medium-rare, or until they start to firm up and are reddish-pink & juicy in the center. Drizzle the pomegranate-port reduction over the chops before serving.

Grilled Garlic and Rosemary Lamb Loin Chops

(Ready in about 2 hours 20 minutes | serving 4|Difficulty: Moderate)

Per serving: Kcal 396, Fat: 36.9g, Net Carbs: 5g, Protein: 12.9g

Ingredients

- Olive oil ½ cup
- Red wine vinegar ¼ cup
- 2 ½ tbsp. Rosemary, minced & fresh
- Lemon ¾ medium, juiced
- Garlic 6 cloves, minced
- Dijon mustard ¾ tsp
- To taste, salt
- 4 lamb leg sirloin chops

Instructions

1. In a big glass or ceramic bowl, combine the olive oil, rosemary, vinegar, lemon juice, mustard, garlic, and salt. Toss in the chops to evenly coat them. Refrigerate for 2 - 4 hours, or overnight, after covering the bowl with plastic wrap.
2. Preheat an outdoor grill to medium-high heat and brush the grate liberally with oil.
3. Shake off any excess marinade from the chops. Remove the remaining marinade and toss it out.
4. Grill the chops for 5 to 7 minutes per side, just until the instant-read thermometer inserted in the center reaches at least 135 degrees F.

Lamb Sliders

(Ready in about 25 minutes | serving 4|Difficulty: Easy)

Per serving: Kcal 459, Fat: 46.1g, Net Carbs: 33.5g, Protein: 28.3g

Ingredients

- Garlic 1 tbsp. Minced
- Cumin ¼ tsp, ground
- Coriander ¼ tsp, ground
- Allspice ¼ tsp ground
- Salt ¼ tsp, or to taste
- Ground lamb 1 lb.
- Black pepper ¼ tsp, or to taste
- Rolls 8 small, split
- Baby spinach 1 cup
- Tzatziki sauce ½ cup
- Red onion ¼ cup, sliced
- Crumbled feta cheese, ¼ cup

Instructions

1. Preheat an outdoor grill to medium-high heat and brush the grate liberally with oil.
2. In a mixing bowl, combine garlic, coriander, allspice, salt, cumin, and pepper; add lamb and toss thoroughly. Make 2-ounce patties out of the mixture.
3. Grill patties for 2 to 3 minutes per side on a hot grill until cooked through. At least 160 degrees F should be read on an instant-read thermometer placed into the center. Place the rolls on the grill & cook for 1 to 2 minutes, or until toasted.
4. To make a slider, layer red onion, tzatziki sauce, spinach, red onion, lamb patty, and feta cheese in each roll.

Lamb Souvlaki

(Ready in about 3 hours 25 minutes | serving 4|Difficulty: Moderate)

Per serving: Kcal 346, Fat: 29.3g, Net Carbs: 1.4g, Protein: 18.8g

Ingredients

- Olive oil ⅓ cup
- Lemon juice 1 ½ tbsp., freshly squeezed
- Red wine vinegar 1 ½ tbsp.
- Black pepper ¼ tsp, ground
- Oregano 1 ½ tbsp., chopped & fresh
- Garlic 2 cloves, minced
- Salt, ½ tsp
- 1 ½ lb. Leg of lamb, boneless & trimmed

Instructions

1. In a medium mixing bowl, combine the olive oil, red wine vinegar, lemon juice, oregano, salt, garlic, and pepper. Stir in the cubed lamb until it is well covered in the marinade. Refrigerate for 3 hours or overnight, covered.
2. Preheat an outdoor grill to medium-high heat and brush the grate liberally with oil.
3. Thread prepared lamb onto skewers using skewers, and store any marinade that remains. Grill skewers for 10 to 12 minutes, occasionally basting with the remaining marinade and rotating to ensure even cooking.

Garlic and Rosemary Grilled Lamb Chops

(Ready in about 25 minutes | serving 4|Difficulty: Easy)

Per serving: Kcal 171.5, Fat: 7.8g, Net Carbs: 0.4g, Protein: 23.2g

Ingredients

- Lamb loin 2 lbs.
- Garlic 4 cloves, minced
- Rosemary 1 tbsp., fresh & chopped
- Black pepper 1/2 tsp
- 1 lemon zest
- Kosher salt 1 1/4 tsp
- Olive oil 1/4 cup

Instructions

1. In a measuring cup, mix the garlic, salt, rosemary, pepper, lemon zest, and olive oil.

2. Drizzle the marinade over lamb chops and turn them over to properly cover them. Refrigerate the chops as little as 1 hour or as long as overnight, covered.

3. Grill the lamb chops for 7-10 minutes on medium heat or until they reach an internal temperature of 135 degrees F.

4. Allow your lamb chops to rest for 5 minutes on a plate covered in aluminum foil before serving.

Indian Style Sheekh Kabab

(Ready in about 2 hours 25 minutes | serving 6|Difficulty: Moderate)

Per serving: Kcal 311, Fat: 22.7g, Net Carbs: 6.2g, Protein: 20.2g

Ingredients

- Lean ground lamb 2 lbs.
- Onions 2 medium, finely chopped
- Mint leaves ½ cup, fresh & finely chopped
- Cilantro ½ cup, finely chopped
- Ginger paste 1 tbsp.
- Paste of green chile 1 tbsp.
- Cumin 2 tsp, ground
- Coriander 2 tsp, ground
- Paprika 2 tsp
- Cayenne pepper 1 tsp
- Salt 2 tsp
- Vegetable oil ¼ cup
- Skewers 8

Instructions

1. Combine ginger paste, ground lamb, mint, onions, cilantro, and Chile paste in a large mixing bowl. Cumin, paprika, coriander, cayenne, and salt are used to season. Put it in the fridge for 2 hours after covering.

2. To make sausages, form handfuls of lamb mixture (approximately 1 cup) around skewers. Ensure that the meat is uniformly spread. Keep refrigerated until ready to grill.

3. Preheat the grill to high.

4. Brush the grill grate with oil and place the kabobs on it. Cook for ten min, or until well cooked, occasionally turning to ensure even browning.

(Ready in about 4 hours 25 minutes | serving 4|Difficulty: Moderate)

Per serving: Kcal 438, Fat: 30.6g, Net Carbs: 12.4g, Protein: 27.6g

Ingredients

- Lamb loin chops 2 lbs.
- Olive oil 2 tbsp.
- Garlic 3 cloves, minced
- Cumin 1 tbsp.
- Mixed herbs 1 tsp
- Black pepper ½ tsp
- Coriander ½ tsp, ground
- Cinnamon ¼ tsp
- Cayenne pepper, 1 pinch
- Salt

For Sauce

- Orange marmalade ¼ cup
- Hot chili flakes 1 pinch
- Rice vinegar ½ tbsp.
- Fresh mint 1 tbsp. Chopped

Instructions

1. In a large mixing bowl, place the lamb chops. Olive oil, cumin, garlic, mixed herbs, coriander, pepper, cinnamon, cayenne, and salt are used to season. Toss until the oil and seasonings are well spread. Cover and store in the refrigerator. Allow at least four hours for marinating.

2. Preheat an outdoor grill to high heat and brush the grate gently with oil. Preheat the grill and place the lamb chops on it. Season the chops with salt and pepper. Grill for 4 to 7 minutes on the first side, based on the size of the chops. About a minute before turning, give the chops a half-turn on the grill. Turn and grill the other side for the next 4 to 7 minutes, or until the desired doneness is reached. An instant-read thermometer placed into the center should read 125 to 130 degrees F for medium-rare. Cover loosely with foil and transfer to the serving dish.

3. In a bowl, place the marmalade. Combine the mint, chili flakes, and rice vinegar in a bowl. Toss it all together thoroughly.

4. Serve the chops with the sauce brushed on top.

Grilled Lamb Chops with Curry, Apple and Raisin Sauce

(Ready in about 1 hour 35 minutes | serving 4|Difficulty: Easy)

Per serving: Kcal 500, Fat: 26.6g, Net Carbs: 50.5g, Protein: 20g

Ingredients

- Butter ¼ cup
- Olive oil 1 tbsp.
- Onion 3 cups, chopped
- Garlic 1 clove, crushed
- Curry powder 2 tbsp., or to taste
- Coriander 1 tbsp. Ground
- Cumin 1 tbsp. Ground
- Salt 2 tsp, or to taste
- White pepper 2 tsp
- Thyme 1 tsp, dried
- Lemon ½, seeded & finely chopped
- Apples 3 cups, chopped
- Applesauce 1 cup
- Dark raisins ⅔ cup
- Golden raisins ⅔ cup
- Water 1 tbsp., if needed
- Lamb chops, 4 ounces

Instructions

1. Melt the butter with the olive oil in a pan over medium heat and sauté the garlic and onions until the onion is transparent about 8 minutes. Combine curry powder, dark raisins, cumin, coriander, salt, thyme, white pepper, lemon, applesauce, and golden raisins in a large mixing bowl. Bring the mixture to a boil, reduce to low heat, cover, and cook for 1 hour, or until the sauce has the thickness of applesauce and the raisins are plump and beginning to break apart. If the sauce becomes too thick, add a tablespoon of water.

2. Preheat an outdoor grill to medium heat and brush the grate gently with oil. Season the lamb chops with salt and pepper.

3. Cook for 3 to 5 minutes per side for medium-rare on the hot grate till the chops are very well, grilled to your required color of pink inside, and show grill marks. A thermometer put into the middle of a chop, without touching the bone, should read around 145 degrees F. Serve the sauce with the lamb chops.

Dale's Lamb

(Ready in about 9 hours 30 minutes | serving 4|Difficulty: Difficult)

Per serving: Kcal 451, Fat: 27.2g, Net Carbs: 17.8g, Protein: 32.4g

Ingredients

- Lemon juice ⅔ cup
- Brown sugar ½ cup
- Dijon mustard ¼ cup
- Soy sauce ¼ cup
- Olive oil ¼ cup
- Garlic 2 cloves, minced
- Ginger root 1 piece, fresh & sliced
- Salt 1 tsp
- Black pepper ½ tsp, ground
- 5 lbs. Lamb leg 1, butterflied

Instructions

1. Mix the lemon juice, Dijon mustard, brown sugar, soy sauce, garlic, olive oil, ginger, pepper, and salt in a mixing bowl. Put the lamb in a small bowl. The lemon juice mixture should be poured over the lamb. Refrigerate for 8 hours or overnight, covered.

2. Heat an outside grill to medium. In a small saucepan, drain the marinade and bring it to a boil. Reduce heat to low and continue to whisk continually until the sauce has slightly thickened.

3. Oil your grill grate lightly. Grill the lamb for 40 to 50 minutes over indirect heat, turning to cook both sides, until it reaches the internal temperature of 145 degrees F. Allow it to cool before slicing and covering with the thicker marinade mixture.

PART 5: FISH AND SEAFOOD

Grilled Shrimp with Shrimp Butter

(Ready in about 30 minutes | serving 4|Difficulty: Easy)

Per serving: Kcal 254, Fat: 20g, Net Carbs: 0g, Protein: 20g

Ingredients

- Butter 6 tbsp., unsalted
- 1/2 cup red onion, finely chopped
- 1 1/2 tsp red pepper, crushed
- Shrimp paste 1 tsp
- Lime juice 1 1/2 tsp
- Salt
- Shrimp 24 large, shelled &deveined
- Black pepper
- Wooden skewers 6
- Assorted sprouts & mint leaves for garnish

Instructions

1. Melt 3 tablespoons butter in a small skillet. Add the onion and simmer until softened. Cook, constantly stirring, for 2 minutes, until the crushed red pepper & shrimp paste are fragrant. Season with salt and lime juice, as well as the leftover 3 tbsp. Of butter. Warm the butter with the shrimp.

2. Preheat the grill or a grill pan. Sprinkle the shrimp with pepper and salt before threading those onto the skewers (don't overcrowd them). Grill for 4 minutes totals over high heat, rotating once until lightly browned and barely cooked through. Transfer to a serving plate and top with the shrimp butter. Serve garnished with mint leaves or sprouts.

Grilled Shrimp with Oregano and Lemon

(Ready in about 1 hour 30 minutes | serving 6|Difficulty: Easy)

Per serving: Kcal 291, Fat: 15g, Net Carbs: 3g, Protein: 35g

Ingredients

- Salted capers 1/2 cup, rinsed
- Oregano leaves 1/2 cup
- Garlic 1 clove, minced
- Olive oil 3/4 cup, extra-virgin
- 1 tsp lemon zest, finely grated
- 3 tbsp. Lemon juice, freshly squeezed
- Black pepper, freshly ground
- Shrimp 2 1/2 lbs., shelled & deveined
- Salt

Instructions

1. Place the oregano leaves, drained capers, and garlic on a cutting board and coarsely slice them. Transfer the mixture to a mixing bowl and whisk in 1/2 cup plus 2 tbsp. Olive oil, as well as the lemon zest and juice. Add a pinch of pepper to the sauce.

2. A grill should be fired up. Mix the shrimp with the leftover 2 tbsp., olive oil and a pinch of salt and pepper in a large mixing bowl. Thread the shrimp into metal skewers, then grill over high temperature for about 3 minutes on each side, rotating once, until lightly charred or cooked through. Transfer the shrimp to a dish when they have been removed from the skewers. Serve with a drizzle of sauce on top.

Grilled Sea Scallops with Corn Salad

(Ready in about 50 minutes | serving 4|Difficulty: Easy)

Per serving: Kcal 495, Fat: 31g, Net Carbs: 33g, Protein: 25g

Ingredients

- Corn 6 ears, shucked
- Grape tomatoes 1 pint, halved
- Sliced Scallions 3, light green & white parts only
- Basil leaves 1/3 cup, finely shredded
- Salt & black pepper
- Shallot 1 small, minced
- Balsamic vinegar 2 tbsp.
- Hot water 2 tbsp.
- Dijon mustard 1 tsp
- Safflower oil 1/4 cup + 3 tbsp.
- Sea scallops 1 1/2 lbs.

Instructions

1. Cook the corn until soft in a big pot of boiling salted water, about 5 minutes. Drain and set aside to cool. Remove the kernels from the corn and place them in a big bowl. Season with pepper and salt, and add the scallions, tomatoes, and basil.

2. Blend the shallot with hot water, vinegar, and mustard in a blender. Slowly drizzle in 6 tablespoons of safflower oil while the mixer is running. Toss the corn salad with the vinaigrette, seasoning it with salt and pepper.

3. Toss the scallops with the leftover 1 tbsp. of oil in a large mixing bowl; season with pepper and salt. A large grill pan should be heated. Add half of the scallops to the pan at a time and cook, flipping once, till browned, about four minutes per batch, over moderately high heat. Serve the corn salad stacked high on plates with the scallops on top.

Grilled Scallops with Honeydew-Avocado Salsa

(Ready in about 30 minutes | serving 4|Difficulty: Easy)

Per serving: Kcal 370, Fat: 13g, Net Carbs: 25g, Protein: 41g

Ingredients

- Lime zest, finely grated
- Lime juice 2 tbsp.
- Olive oil, 1 tbsp.
- Honeydew melon 1 1/2 lbs., rind removed & sliced
- Hass avocado 1, sliced into ¼ inch dice
- Salt & black pepper
- Sea scallops 2 lbs.

Instructions

1. Preheat the grill. Combine the lime juice and zest with 1 tbsp. Olive oil in a large mixing bowl. Fold in the diced avocado and honeydew melon using a rubber spatula. Season the salsa with black pepper and salt.

2. Season the scallops with pepper and salt after drizzling them with olive oil. Cook for 3 to 4 minutes per side over high heat, flipping once, until well charred and slightly cooked through. Transfer the scallops to bowls and serve with the salsa on the side.

Grilled Oysters with Spiced Tequila Butter

(Ready in about 25 minutes | serving 4|Difficulty: Easy)
Per serving: Kcal 146, Fat: 14g, Net Carbs: 2.9g, Protein: 3.3g

Ingredients

- Fennel seeds 1/2 tsp
- Red pepper 1/4 tsp, crushed
- Butter 7 tbsp., unsalted
- Sage leaves 1/4 cup, plus for garnish
- Dried oregano 1 tsp
- 2 tbsp. Lemon juice, freshly squeezed
- Tequila 2 tbsp.
- For serving: rock salt
- Kosher salt
- Medium oysters 3 dozen, scrubbed

Instructions

1. Toast the crushed red pepper and fennel seeds in a pan over moderate heat for 1 minute or until fragrant. Place in a mortar and set aside to cool completely. To make a coarse powder, pound the spices in a pestle and transfer them to a dish.
2. Cook 3 1/2 tbsp. Butter in the same skillet over medium heat until it begins to brown, about 2 minutes. Cook for 2 minutes, rotating once until the sage is crisp. Place the sage on the plate with a slotted spoon. Pour the browned butter into the spice bowl. Repeat with remaining butter and 36 sage leaves, setting aside the leaves for garnish.
3. Crush the very first batch of the fried sage leaves with the pestle in the mortar. Season with salt and pepper, then add the crushed sage, lemon juice, oregano, and tequila to the butter.
4. Fire up the grill. Using rock salt, coat a platter. Grill the oysters over high heat, flat side up, for 1 to 2 minutes, or until they open. Remove the oysters from the flat top shell and set them on the rock salt, being cautious not to leak their fluid. Serve the oysters with warm tequila butter and a crisp sage leaf on top.

Grilled Oysters with Chorizo Butter

(Ready in about 45 minutes | serving 6|Difficulty: Easy)
Per serving: Kcal 61, Fat: 5.1g, Net Carbs: 1.5g, Protein: 2.5g

Ingredients

- Mexican chorizo 4 ounces, fresh & casings removed
- Butter 1 1/2 sticks, unsalted
- Lime juice 2 tbsp. Fresh
- Salt
- 18 large oysters (Louisiana), scrubbed
- Cilantro leaves
- Lime zest, finely grated for garnish

Instructions

1. Cook the chorizo in a skillet over medium heat, breaking up with a spoon until lightly browned, about 8 minutes. Allow cooling in a bowl before breaking into small clumps.
2. In a small skillet, add 1 tbsp. of water and bring to a low simmer. Add a few cubes of butter to the skillet, stirring till melted before adding more. Season with salt and pepper after adding the lime juice chorizo. Keep warm on a low heat setting.
3. Preheat the grill. Place the oysters' flat side up on the grill. Grill the shells over high temperatures until they begin to open slightly. Carefully transfer to a plate and remove the top shell with cooking gloves or a mitt. Garnish the oysters with chorizo butter and cilantro leaves, as well as lime zest. Serve immediately.

Citrus-Soy Squid

(Ready in about 45 minutes | serving 4|Difficulty: Easy)

Per serving: Kcal 0.12, Fat: 0g, Net Carbs: 0.02g, Protein: 0g

Ingredients

- Mirin 1 cup
- Soy sauce 1 cup
- Lemon juice 1/3 cup, fresh
- Water 2 cups
- Squid tentacles 2 lbs. Left whole, bodies cut crosswise

Instructions

1. Combine the mirin, yuzu juice, soy sauce, and water in a mixing bowl.
2. Refrigerate half of the marinade in an airtight container for later use. Add the squid to a bowl with the leftover marinade and set aside for at least 30 min or up to 4 hours at room temperature.
3. Preheat the grill. The squid should be drained. Grill for 3 minutes over moderately high heat, rotating once, till tender and white throughout. Serve immediately.

Grilled Lobsters with Miso-Chile Butter

(Ready in about 40 minutes | serving 6|Difficulty: Easy)

Per serving: Kcal 336, Fat: 12.3g, Net Carbs: 47.1g, Protein: 6g

Ingredients

- Butter 1 stick, unsalted & cubed
- White miso 2 tbsp.
- Sriracha 1 tbsp.
- Lemon juice 2 tbsp.
- For serving, wedges
- Scallions 2 bunches
- Canola oil 1 tbsp.
- Pepper
- Kosher salt
- Metal skewers, 8 long
- Claws detached 4 lobsters 1 ½ lb., halved lengthwise

Instructions

1. Melt the butter in a small saucepan. Combine the Sriracha, miso, and lemon juice in a mixing bowl. 1/4 cup miso-Chile butter is set aside for serving.
2. Preheat the grill. Mix the scallions with the oil in a large mixing bowl and season with pepper and salt. 5 minutes over moderate heat, rotating once until faintly browned and tender. Toss 1 tbsp. of the miso-Chile butter with the scallions.
3. To keep the lobster bodies straight, skewer them from the tail to head. two tbsp. miso-Chile butter, brushed over lobster meat Turn and bast the lobster claws and bodies with the leftover miso-Chile butter over moderate heat until the shells are red, 8 to 10 mins for the tails or 12 to 15 mins for the claws.
4. Arrange the scallions on top of the lobsters on a tray or plates. Serve over lemon wedges as well as the 1/4 cup miso-Chile butter that was set aside.

Grilled Oysters with Spicy Tarragon Butter

(Ready in about 40 minutes | serving 4|Difficulty: Easy)

Per serving: Kcal 390, Fat: 27g, Net Carbs: 3g, Protein: 2g

Ingredients

- 2 sticks butter, 1/2 lbs. Unsalted & softened
- Tarragon 3 tbsp. Chopped
- Hot sauce 2 tbsp.
- Kosher salt 1/2 tsp
- 1/4 tsp pepper, freshly ground
- Oysters 3 dozen, such as gulf coast

Instructions

1. Preheat the grill. Pulse the butter, hot sauce, tarragon, pepper, and salt in a food processor until smooth. Roll the tarragon butter into a 2-inch-thick log using a sheet of plastic wrap. Refrigerate the butter for about 15 minutes or until it is slightly firm. Cut the butter in 36 parts with a knife.

2. Place the oyster's flat-side up on the heated grill. Cover the grill, then cook for 5 minutes, or until the oysters open. Place the oysters on a tray with tongs, attempting to keep the liquor within. Remove the top shells as soon as possible, and dislodge the oysters from the bottom shells. Transfer the oysters to the grill with the pat of tarragon butter on top of each. Cover the grill and heat for 1 minute, till the butter is mostly melted as well as the oysters are heated. Serve immediately.

Grilled Scallops with Mexican Corn Salad

(Ready in about 40 minutes | serving 4|Difficulty: Easy)

Per serving: Kcal 220, Fat: 24g, Net Carbs: 35g, Protein: 12.7g

Ingredients

- Minced Garlic 1 clove
- 1 tbsp. Red onion, minced
- Lime juice 2 tbsp. Fresh
- Corn ears 8, husked
- For brushing vegetable oil
- Mayonnaise 1/3 cup
- Chile powder 1 tsp
- 1 ¼ ounce ricotta Salata cheese 4 ounces, crumbled
- Salt & black pepper
- Hot sauce
- Sea scallops, 12 large
- For serving, lime wedges

Instructions

1. Preheat the grill. Toss the onion and garlic with lime juice in a large mixing dish and set aside for 10 minutes.

2. Brush the corn using oil, grill over medium heat for about 10 minutes, or until charred or just tender. Cut the kernels off cobs and transfer them to a work surface.

3. In a mixing bowl, combine the onion, garlic, and lime juice with the mayonnaise and chili powder. Toss the corn and cheese into the bowl. Salt, pepper, and hot sauce can all be used to season the dish.

4. Season the scallops with salt and black pepper after brushing them with vegetable oil. Grill for 2-3 minutes per side over high temperature until well browned and slightly cooked through. Serve the corn salad on 4 plates with the scallops on top. Serve over lime wedges on the side.

Pop-Open Clams with Horseradish-Tabasco Sauce

(Ready in about 15 minutes | serving 4|Difficulty: Easy)

Per serving: Kcal 134, Fat: 8g, Net Carbs: 5g, Protein: 9g

Ingredients

- Unsalted butter 4 tbsp., softened
- Horseradish 2 tbsp. Drained
- Tabasco 1 tbsp.
- Lemon zest 1/4 tsp, finely grated
- Lemon juice 1 tbsp. Fresh
- Pimentón de la vera 1/4 tsp, sweet
- Salt
- Littleneck clams 2 dozen, scrubbed
- Crusty white bread grilled slices, for serving

Instructions

1. Preheat the grill. Combine the butter, Tabasco, horseradish, lemon juice, lemon zest, and pimentón de la Vera in a small bowl. Season with salt and pepper.

2. Grill the clams over medium temperature for about 25 seconds or until they pop open. Carefully flip the clams over so that the meat side is down, using tongs. Cook for another 20 seconds, or until the clam fluids begin to simmer. Place the clams in a serving bowl and set them aside. Serve with grilled bread and roughly 1/2 teaspoon horseradish-Tabasco sauce on top of each clam.

Shrimp and Scallops with Lemony Soy

(Ready in about 30 minutes | serving 8|Difficulty: Easy)

Per serving: Kcal 139, Fat: 5.6g, Net Carbs: 4.9g, Protein: 16.7g

Ingredients

- 1 1/2 cups soy sauce, low-sodium
- Mirin 1 cup
- Sake 1 cup
- Lemons 2, sliced
- Jalapeños 2, thinly sliced
- Medium shrimp 1 lb., shelled & deveined
- Sea scallops 1 lb. Large
- For grilling vegetable oil

Instructions

1. Combine the soy sauce, sake, mirin, lemon slices, and jalapenos in a ceramic baking dish.

2. Thread the shrimp onto eight bamboo skewers and place them in the marinade, twisting to evenly coat them. The scallops should be done in the same manner. Drain the seafood after 30 minutes in the refrigerator, turning once halfway through.

3. Grates should be oiled, and a grill should be lighted. Brush the scallops and shrimp with oil and cook until gently browned, about 4 minutes, flipping once or twice. Serve immediately.

Shrimp and Lemon Skewers with Feta-Dill Sauce

(Ready in about 30 minutes | serving 4|Difficulty: Easy)

Per serving: Kcal 378, Fat: 42g, Net Carbs: 32g, Protein: 11g

Ingredients

- 1/2 cup yogurt, plain & low fat
- Sliced scallion 1, light green & white parts only
- Finely chopped, garlic 4 cloves
- 2 1/2 tbsp. Dill, finely chopped

- 2 ounces crumbled feta cheese, 1/2 cup
- Salt & black pepper
- 1/4 cup olive oil, extra-virgin
- Peeled & deveined large shrimp, 2 lbs.
- Lemons 2, each sliced into 12 wedges

Instructions

1. Preheat the grill. Combine the yogurt, 1/4 tsp garlic, scallion, and 1/2 tbsp. Dill in a medium mixing bowl. Mix in the feta, softly mashing it in. Add salt & pepper to taste.

2. Combine the leftover minced garlic and 2 tbsp. Dill with the olive oil in a large mixing bowl. Season with pepper and salt and toss to coat the shrimp and lemons on each of the 12 skewers, thread four shrimp with 2 lemon wedges. Season with pepper and salt and cook, occasionally turning, over a medium-hot heat till the shrimp are charred as well as cooked through, about five minutes. Transfer the skewers to a plate and top with the feta sauce right away.

Grilled Scallops with Honeydew-Avocado Salsa

(Ready in about 30 minutes | serving 4|Difficulty: Easy)

Per serving: Kcal 370, Fat: 13g, Net Carbs: 25g, Protein: 41g

Ingredients

- Lime zest, Finely grated
- Lime juice 2 tbsp.
- 1 tbsp. Olive oil, extra-virgin, plus for grilling

- Honeydew melon 1 1/2 lbs., rind removed & sliced
- Hass avocado 1, sliced into 1/4-inch dice
- Salt & black pepper
- Sea scallops 2 lbs. Large

Instructions

1. Preheat the grill. Combine the lime juice and zest with 1 tablespoon olive oil in a large mixing bowl. Fold in the diced avocado and honeydew melon using a rubber spatula. Season the salsa with black pepper and salt.

2. Season the scallops with black pepper and salt after drizzling them with olive oil. Cook for 3 - 4 minutes per side over high heat, flipping once, until well charred and slightly cooked through. Place the scallops on plates and serve with the salsa on the side.

Greek Grilled Scallop Sandwiches

(Ready in about 30 minutes | serving 4|Difficulty: Easy)

Per serving: Kcal 465, Fat: 26g, Net Carbs: 18g, Protein: 40g

Ingredients

- Greek-style yogurt, 1/4 cup
- Saffron threads 1 pinch, crumbled
- Rice vinegar 1 1/2 tsp
- Sea salt & black pepper
- Black plum 1 small, thinly sliced
- Olive oil (Extra-virgin)
- 1 ¼ lb. Sea scallops 12 large
- Prosciutto 2 slices, cut into strips
- 1 cup pea tendrils 36

Instructions

1. Preheat the grill. Combine the saffron, yogurt, and vinegar in a mixing bowl and season with pepper and salt.

2. Coat the plum slices with oil, then grill for 30 seconds per side over high heat until gently charred. Sprinkle the scallops with oil, salt, and pepper, grill them over medium temperature for about 1 minute per side, or until charred or just cooked through.

3. Each scallop should be cut in half crosswise. On the bottom half of each scallop, place a plum slice. Place the prosciutto strips on top of the plums, top with two pea tendrils and the scallop tops. Place 3 toothpicks on each dish and secure with toothpicks. 1 tsp of the yogurt sauce should be spread on each scallop sandwich, and the leftover pea tendrils should be garnished. Serve with a drizzle of olive oil and a pinch of salt.

Spiced Crab Tacos

(Ready in about 25 minutes | serving 4|Difficulty: Easy)

Per serving: Kcal 200, Fat: 12g, Net Carbs: 13g, Protein: 11g

Ingredients

- Tomatoes 2 medium, finely chopped
- Red radishes 2 large, sliced into ¼ inch dice
- Red onion 1/2 small, finely chopped
- 1/4 cup cilantro, chopped
- Sriracha Chile sauce 2 tsp
- Salt
- Jalapeño 1 large
- Bell pepper 1/2 red, sliced into 1/3-inch pieces
- Bell pepper 1/2 yellow, sliced into 1/3-inch pieces
- Olive oil 3 tbsp., extra-virgin
- Lime juice 1 tbsp. Fresh
- Chopped mint 1 tbsp.
- Lump crabmeat ½ lbs.
- 8 flour tortillas (10 inches), halved

Instructions

1. Combine the radishes, tomatoes, 2 tbsp. Cilantro, red onion, and Sriracha in a medium mixing bowl. Using salt, season the salsa.

2. Preheat the grill. Over medium heat, turn the jalapeno until it is charred all over. Allow it cool completely before discarding the charred skin, stem, and seeds. Chop the jalapeno finely.

3. Combine the jalapeno, yellow and red bell peppers, lime juice, olive oil, mint, and the leftover 2 tbsp. Cilantro in a medium mixing bowl. Season with salt and carefully fold in the crabmeat.

4. Grill the tortillas for about twenty seconds per side over high heat or until charred and puffed in spots. Warm tortillas & salsa are served with the spicy crab.

Grilled Shrimp with Miso Butter

(Ready in about 30 minutes | serving 4|Difficulty: Easy)

Per serving: Kcal 190, Fat: 8g, Net Carbs: 2g, Protein: 23g

Ingredients

- 1 stick butter, unsalted & softened
- White miso 2 tbsp.
- 1/2 tsp lemon zest, finely grated
- Lemon juice 1 tbsp. Fresh
- 1 tbsp. Scallion, thinly sliced plus more for garnish
- Shelled & deveined shrimp 1 lb.
- Canola oil 2 tbsp.
- Minced garlic 1 clove
- Chile powder 1 tsp
- Kosher salt 1 tsp
- Pickled mustard seeds 1 1/2 tsp

Instructions

1. Puree the butter with lemon zest, miso, and lemon juice in a food processor until smooth. Pulse in the 1 tbsp. of scallion until it is all mixed. Set aside the miso butter in a large mixing dish.

2. Mix the shrimp with the garlic, oil, Chile powder, and salt in a separate large mixing dish and set aside for 10 minutes.

3. Preheat the grill. Grill the shrimp over high temperature, turning once, for about 4 minutes, or until just cooked through. Toss the shrimp in the miso butter immediately until fully coated. Serve the shrimp garnished with scallions, pickled mustard seeds, and brine.

Pineapple Shrimp Skewers

(Ready in about 35 minutes | serving 4|Difficulty: Easy)
Per serving: Kcal 223.8, Fat: 2.2g, Net Carbs: 28g, Protein: 24.3g
Ingredients

- Pineapple 3 cups, cubed
- Shrimp 1 pound, peeled & deveined
- Olive oil 3 tbsp., extra-virgin
- Sweet chili sauce 3 tbsp.
- Garlic 2 cloves, minced
- 2 tsp. Ginger, freshly grated
- 2 tsp. Sesame oil, toasted
- Red pepper flakes, crushed
- Red pepper flakes 1/2 tsp., crushed
- Kosher salt
- For garnish, sesame seeds
- Green onions Thinly sliced for garnish
- For serving, Lime wedges

Instructions

1. Preheat the grill to medium and soak the wooden skewers in water. Using skewers, alternate between shrimp and pineapple until all are used, then put on a large baking sheet.
2. Combine sesame oil, olive oil, garlic, chili sauce, ginger, sesame oil, & red pepper flakes in a medium mixing bowl and season with salt. Brush all over the skewers with the mixture that has been whisked together.
3. Arrange skewers on the grill, then cook for 4 to 6 minutes, turning once, till shrimp is cooked through.
4. Before serving, garnish with green onions and sesame seeds.

Grilled Shrimp Foil Packets

(Ready in about 25 minutes | serving 4|Difficulty: Easy)
Per serving: Kcal 527, Fat: 14.3g, Net Carbs: 62g, Protein: 48g
Ingredients

- Shrimp 1 1/2 lb. , peeled & deveined
- Minced Garlic 2 cloves
- Thinly sliced Andouille sausages 2
- Corn 2 ears
- 1 lb. Red bliss potatoes, cut into 1-inch pieces
- 2 tbsp. Olive oil (extra-virgin)
- Old bay (seasoning) 1 tbsp.
- Kosher salt & black pepper
- 2 tbsp. Parsley, freshly chopped
- Butter 4 tbsp.
- Lemon 1, sliced

Instructions

1. Preheat the grill to high heat. Cut four 12-inch-long sheets of foil. Over the foil sheets, evenly distribute the shrimp, sausage, garlic, corn, and potatoes. Drizzle with oil, then season with Old Bay seasoning plus salt and pepper to taste. To combine, gently toss everything together. Each mixture should be topped with parsley, lemon, and a tbsp. of butter.
2. To properly cover the food, fold the foil packs crosswise over the shrimp boil mixture. To seal the top and bottom edges, roll them together.
3. Place foil packs on the grill and cook for 15 - 20 minutes, or until just cooked through.

Perfect Grilled Fish

(Ready in about 15 minutes | serving 4|Difficulty: Easy)

Per serving: Kcal 123, Fat: 25.5g, Net Carbs: 0.31g, Protein: 1.3g

Ingredients

- Chili powder 1 tsp.
- Oregano 1 tsp., dried
- Cayenne pepper 1/4 tsp.
- Kosher salt
- Black pepper, freshly ground
- ½ inch thick fillet white fish, such as cod
- For serving, lime wedges

Instructions

1. Preheat the grill to high heat. Combine chili powder, cayenne, oregano, and salt and pepper in a mixing bowl.
2. Season the fish with spice mixture all over.
3. Cook for 8 - 10 minutes, skin-side down, until almost completely opaque throughout.
4. Cook for another 2 to 3 minutes on the other side, or until opaque throughout.

Grilled Halibut

(Ready in about 20 minutes | serving 4|Difficulty: Easy)

Per serving: Kcal 150, Fat: 3g, Net Carbs: 0g, Protein: 28g

Ingredients

For the halibut

- 4 halibut steaks 6-oz.
- 2 tbsp. Olive oil (extra-virgin)
- Kosher salt & black pepper

For the mango salsa

- Mango 1, diced
- Pepper 1 red, finely chopped
- Onion 1/2 red, diced
- Jalapeno 1, minced
- 1 tbsp. Cilantro, freshly chopped
- 1 lime juice

Instructions

1. Preheat the grill to moderate temperature and spray both sides of the halibut with oil before seasoning with pepper and salt.
2. Cook five minutes per side on the grill until halibut is cooked through.
3. To make salsa, follow these steps: Combine all ingredients and add salt and pepper in a medium mixing bowl. Serve the salsa with halibut.

Lemony Grilled Salmon

(Ready in about 20 minutes | serving 4|Difficulty: Easy)

Per serving: Kcal 270, Fat: 11.5g, Net Carbs: 14.2g, Protein: 28g

Ingredients

- Skin-on 4 salmon fillets (6-oz.)
- Olive oil (Extra-virgin) for brushing
- Kosher salt & black pepper
- Lemons 2, sliced
- Butter 2 tbsp.

Instructions

1. Preheat the grill to high heat. Season the salmon with pepper and salt after brushing it with oil. Grill the lemon slices and salmon for 5 minutes per side, or until the salmon is cooked completely and the lemons are charred.

2. Top the salmon with a pat of butter and grilled lemons as soon as it comes off the grill.

Foil Pack Grilled Salmon with Lemony Asparagus

(Ready in about 20 minutes | serving 4|Difficulty: Easy)

Per serving: Kcal 360, Fat: 9g, Net Carbs: 4g, Protein: 36g

Ingredients

- Asparagus spears 20, trimmed
- Skin-on 4 salmon fillets (6-oz)
- Butter 4 tbsp. , divided
- Lemons 2, sliced
- Kosher salt & black pepper
- For garnish, fresh dill

Instructions

1. On a flat surface, place 2 pieces of foil. Top five asparagus spears with 1 tbsp. Butter, salmon fillet, and two lemon slices on foil. Wrap the remaining ingredients loosely, then repeat till you have 4 packets total.

2. High heat the grill. Place the foil packets on the grill and cook for 10 minutes, or until the salmon is done and the asparagus is tender.

3. Serve with dill as a garnish.

Grilled Salmon with Mango Salsa

(Ready in about 25 minutes | serving 4|Difficulty: Easy)

Per serving: Kcal 79, Fat: 1g, Net Carbs: 19g, Protein: 2g

Ingredients

- 4 salmon fillets (6 ounces)
- Garlic powder 1 tsp
- Chili powder 1 tsp
- Pepper & salt to taste
- 1 lime juice

For Mango Salsa

- Mangoes 3, diced
- Red pepper ½, diced
- Red onion ½, diced
- Jalapeño 1 small, seeded & finely chopped
- Cilantro leaves ¼ cup, roughly chopped

Instructions

1. Combine mangos, onions, red peppers, jalapenos, and cilantro in a medium mixing bowl. Keep it aside until you're ready to use it.
2. Combine garlic powder, salt, chili powder, and pepper in a mixing bowl. Fillets of salmon should be rubbed with the mixture. Grill for 7-8 mins over medium heat.
3. Serve by squeezing fresh lime juice overcooked fish and topping with mango salsa.

Easy Grilled Mahi with Avocado and Corn Salsa

(Ready in about 25 minutes | serving 4|Difficulty: Easy)

Per serving: Kcal 227, Fat: 11g, Net Carbs: 25g, Protein: 10g

Ingredients

- Mahi Mahi fillets 4, thawed
- Olive oil 2 tbsp.
- Cumin 2 tsp, ground
- Chili powder 2 tsp
- Salt ½ tsp
- Pepper ¼ tsp

For Corn Salsa

- Corn ears 2, shucked & removed
- Poblano pepper 1 small, seeded & chopped

- Ripe avocado 1, cubed
- Red pepper 1/2 cup, chopped
- Purple onion 1/3 cup, chopped
- Olive oil 3 tbsp.
- Sugar 1 tbsp.
- Vinegar 1 tbsp.
- Salt 1/2 tsp
- Pepper 1/4 tsp

Instructions

For the Salsa

1. In a large mixing bowl, combine all of the ingredients. While the fish is grilling, chill it.

For Mahi

1. Preheat an outdoor grill to medium-high temperature.
2. Combine olive oil, chili powder, cumin, salt, and pepper in a small dish.
3. Rub to Mahi fillets (uncooked) using a brush.
4. Grill for 4 mins (depending on the thickness of a fillet) or until the fish flakes easily and the internal temperature reaches 145 degrees F.
5. Serve with a dollop of salsa.

Grilled Shrimp with Oregano and Lemon

(Ready in about 1 hour 30 minutes | serving 6|Difficulty: Easy)

Per serving: Kcal 291, Fat: 15g, Net Carbs: 3g, Protein: 35g

Ingredients

- Salted capers ½ cup
- Oregano leaves ½ cup
- Garlic 1 clove
- 3/4 cup olive oil (extra-virgin)
- 1 tsp. Lemon zest, finely grated
- 3 tbsp. Lemon juice, freshly squeezed
- Black pepper, freshly ground
- Shrimp 2 1/2 lb.
- Salt

Instructions

1.   Place the drained capers, oregano leaves, and garlic on a cutting board and coarsely slice them. Transfer the mixture to a mixing bowl and add 1/2 cup + 2 tbsp. Olive oil, as well as the lemon zest and juice. Season the sauce with a pinch of black pepper.

2.   Preheat the grill. Mix the shrimp with the leftover 2 tbsp. Of olive oil in a large mixing dish and season lightly with pepper and salt. Thread the shrimp into metal skewers, grill over high heat, flipping once, for 3 minutes per side, or until lightly browned and cooked through. Transfer the shrimp to a plate after removing them from the skewers. Serve with a dollop of sauce on top.

Grilled Salmon with Creamy Pesto Sauce

(Ready in about 20 minutes | serving 4|Difficulty: Easy)

Per serving: Kcal 351, Fat: 25.4g, Net Carbs: 3.1g, Protein: 28g

Ingredients

- Salmon fillets 4
- Salt 1/4 tsp.
- Pepper 1/4 tsp.
- Olive oil 2 tbsp.
- Milk ¼ cup
- Philadelphia cream cheese 4 oz.
- Pesto 2 tbsp.
- Fresh parsley 1 tbsp.

Instructions

1.   Preheat the grill to medium.

2.   Brush the fish on both sides with oil and season with pepper and salt. Grill for 10 minutes, skin-side down, or till fish flakes easily with the fork.

3.   Meanwhile, stir while cooking cream cheese and milk in a saucepan over medium heat for 2 to 3 minutes, or till cream cheese is fully melted and sauce is thoroughly combined. Add the pesto and mix well.

4.   Serve the fish with the sauce and parsley on top.

Grilled Calamari with Minted Red Pepper

(Ready in about 40 minutes | serving 4|Difficulty: Easy)

Per serving: Kcal 240, Fat: 15g, Net Carbs: 10g, Protein: 19g

Ingredients

- Garlic 1 clove
- 2 1/2 tbsp. Olive oil (extra-virgin)
- Kosher salt 3 1/4 tsp.
- 10 small calamari 1 lb.
- Red bell peppers 3 large
- Sherry vinegar 2 tsp.
- Fresh mint leaves 10

Instructions

2. In a large mixing bowl, grate garlic. Add 3 tbsp. salt and 1 tbsp. olive oil. Toss in the calamari to coat. Refrigerate for ten min or up to two hours in the refrigerator.

3. Preheat the grill to high. Using olive oil, lightly coat the peppers. Grill for 20 minutes, rotating once or twice until charred evenly. Cover with plastic wrap once transferred to a bowl. Remove the plastic with care and set it aside to cool slightly. Scrape off the skin quickly and gently. Remove the cores and seeds from the peppers, reserving the juices. Using a 1-inch-wide strip cutter, cut into 1-inch-wide strips. Combine peppers, vinegar, 1 tbsp. olive oil, juices, and 1/4 tsp salt in a mixing bowl.

4. Grill calamari for 1 minute per side over high heat, until lightly charred. Cooking juices should be shaken out. Toss the mint into the pepper mixture and place it on a serving platter. Serve with calamari on top, seasoning to taste and a drizzle of 1/2 tbsp. olive oil.

Tuna Niçoise Burgers

(Ready in about 30 minutes | serving 4|Difficulty: Easy)

Per serving: Kcal 900, Fat: 67g, Net Carbs: 13g, Protein: 55g

Ingredients

- Fresh tuna 1 1/4 lb.
- Scallions 2
- Kalamata olives, 12 pitted
- Salted capers 1 tbsp.
- Salt
- Black pepper, freshly ground
- Olive oil (extra-virgin)
- Mayonnaise 1/4 cup
- Tomatoes, sliced
- Anchovy paste 1 1/2 tsp.
- Brioche buns 4
- Arugula

Instructions

1. Freeze for 5 minutes after spreading tuna, olives, scallions, and capers on a plate. Pulse the tuna in a food processor until it is finely chopped. Season with pepper and salt after transferring the mixture to a bowl. Make four 4-inch patties out of the mixture.

2. Preheat the grill or a grill pan. Sprinkle the burgers with olive oil, then grill over moderate to high heat, rotating once, for about 6 minutes, or until golden and crispy and just cooked through.

3. Combine the anchovy paste and mayonnaise in a bowl; place on the buns. Close the burger and serve with the tomato and arugula.

(Ready in about 35 minutes | serving 4|Difficulty: Easy)

Per serving: Kcal 369, Fat: 18g, Net Carbs: 7g, Protein: 42g[OBJ]

Ingredients

- Olive oil 1/4 cup
- Garlic 1 clove
- Dried sage 1/2 tsp
- Dried rosemary 1/2 tsp
- Wine vinegar 2 tbsp.
- Salt 1/2 tsp.
- 1/4 tsp. Black pepper, freshly ground
- 2 lbs. Trout fillets 8

Instructions

1. Heat the grill at high. Combine the oil, sage, garlic, and rosemary in a small pan. Cook, occasionally stirring, for about 2 minutes, or until the garlic begins to brown. Remove the pan from the heat and add the 1/4 tsp salt, vinegar, and pepper immediately.

2. In a large stainless steel pan, place the trout fillets. The leftover 1/4 teaspoon salt should be sprinkled on the trout. Half of the vinegar and oil mixture should be added and turned to coat. Cook the trout for 2 minutes with the skin side down on the grill. Cook for another 2 minutes for 1/4-inch-thick fillets, or until just done. Pour the remaining vinegar and oil mixture over the hot trout before serving.

PART 5: VEGETABLE RECIPES

Grilled Mexican Street Corn (Elote)

(Ready in about 30 minutes | serving 4|Difficulty: Easy)

Per serving: Kcal 201, Fat: 9g, Net Carbs: 30g, Protein: 7g

Ingredients

- For brushing, Vegetable oil
- 4 corn ears, husked
- Kosher salt 1/2 tsp
- 1/2 tsp black pepper, freshly ground
- Chipotle mayonnaise 1/4 cup
- 1/4 cup Cotija cheese, grated fresh

Instructions

1. Heat a grill to medium-high. Oil the grill grate. Season corn with pepper and salt after lightly brushing it with oil. Grill for 4 - 5 minutes per side over a covered grill until cooked and thoroughly charred. Allow cooling slightly before serving. Serve with mayonnaise and cheese.

Grilled Mushroom Antipasto Salad

(Ready in about 40 minutes | serving 4|Difficulty: Easy)

Per serving: Kcal 79, Fat: 7g, Net Carbs: 3.1g, Protein: 2g

Ingredients

- Mushrooms 2 lb.
- 7 tbsp. Olive oil (extra-virgin), divided
- Kosher salt
- 2 tbsp. White wine vinegar
- 1 tsp. Pepper (Aleppo-style)
- 1 tsp. Oregano, dried
- Finely grated, garlic 1 clove
- Black pepper, freshly ground
- Parmesan 2 oz., shaved
- Castelvetrano olives ½ cup, coarsely chopped
- ¼ cup peppadew peppers, drained & coarsely chopped

Instructions

2. Heat a grill to high temperatures. In a large mixing bowl, toss the mushrooms with 3 tbsp. of oil to coat. Grill for 2–6 minutes, occasionally flipping with tongs until lightly charred. Season with salt and return to the bowl.

3. In a separate bowl, whisk together the vinegar, oregano, Aleppo-style pepper, garlic, and the remaining 4 tbsp. oil; season with pepper and salt. Toss the mushrooms in the sauce to coat them. Toss in the olives, Parmesan, and Peppadew peppers until well mixed.

Grilled Green Beans

(Ready in about 20 minutes | serving 4|Difficulty: Easy)

Per serving: Kcal 28, Fat: 0.5g, Net Carbs: 5.6g, Protein: 1.4g

Ingredients

- Green beans 1 lb. , ends trimmed
- 3 tbsp. Olive oil (extra-virgin)
- Soy sauce 2 tbsp.
- Chili garlic paste 1 tbsp.
- Honey 2 tsp.
- Red pepper flakes 1 pinch
- Kosher salt

For garnish

- Sesame seeds
- Green onions, thinly sliced
- Chopped Roasted peanuts

Instructions

1. Preheat a medium-high grill pan. Combine the oil, soy sauce, honey, chili garlic paste, and red pepper flakes in a large mixing bowl, then toss in the green beans to coat. Add salt and pepper to taste.
2. Put green beans onto grill pan, heat for about 7 minutes, or until charred all over.
3. Green onions, sesame seeds, and peanuts can be added as garnishes.

Best-Ever Grilled Potatoes

(Ready in about 20 minutes | serving 4|Difficulty: Easy)

Per serving: Kcal 278, Fat: 11.8g, Net Carbs: 40g, Protein: 4.8g

Ingredients

- Russet potatoes 4 large, sliced into wedges
- Garlic powder 2 tsp.
- Kosher salt 1 tsp.
- 1 tsp. Black pepper, freshly ground
- 1/2 c. Olive oil (extra-virgin)
- 2 tbsp. Herbs, freshly chopped such as parsley

Instructions

1. Bring a pot of salted water to a boil, add the potatoes and cook for 5 to 7 minutes, or until al dente. Drain and set aside to cool.
2. Preheat the grill to moderate and lightly oil the grates. Combine garlic powder, pepper, and salt in a large mixing bowl, then toss in olive oil. Toss in the potatoes lightly to coat. Remove the potatoes from the oil and set aside any remaining oil in a bowl.
3. Cook for 5 minutes on the grill, turning once, until golden brown.
4. Return the potatoes to the leftover oil mixture and toss them one more.

Grilled Asparagus

(Ready in about 10 minutes | serving 4|Difficulty: Easy)

Per serving: Kcal 45, Fat: 3g, Net Carbs: 3.9g, Protein: 2.2g

Ingredients

- Asparagus 2 lb. , stalks trimmed
- 2 tbsp. Olive oil (extra-virgin)
- Kosher salt & black pepper

Instructions

1. Over high heat, preheat a grill. Season asparagus liberally with pepper and salt after lightly tossing it in oil.
2. Cook for 3 to 4 minutes on the grill, regularly flipping, until tender and charred.

Grilled Balsamic Mushrooms

(Ready in about 35 minutes | serving 4|Difficulty: Easy)

Per serving: Kcal 45, Fat: 0g, Net Carbs: 9g, Protein: 3g

Ingredients

- Balsamic vinegar 1/4 cup
- 2 tbsp. Soy sauce (low-sodium)
- Garlic 2 cloves, minced
- Black pepper, freshly ground
- Cremini mushrooms 1 lb. , sliced
- Parsley, freshly chopped for garnish

Instructions

1. Whisk together the balsamic vinegar, garlic, soy sauce, and pepper in a large mixing bowl. Add the mushrooms and let them marinate for 20 minutes. While the mushrooms marinate, immerse wooden skewers in water.
2. Preheat the grill to medium-high heat. Grill mushrooms on skewers for 2 - 3 minutes per side.
3. Before serving, garnish with parsley.

Veggie Kabobs

(Ready in about 45 minutes | serving 4|Difficulty: Easy)

Per serving: Kcal 128, Fat: 7g, Net Carbs: 15g, Protein: 5g

Ingredients

- Zucchini 2 medium, sliced into 1 inch thick pieces
- 1 package mushrooms (10 oz.) Cleaned & halved
- Red onion 1 medium, cut into wedges
- Lemons 2 small, cut into eighths
- 3 tbsp. Olive oil (extra-virgin)
- Garlic 1 clove, grated
- 1 tsp. Thyme, freshly chopped
- Red pepper flakes 1 Pinch, crushed
- Kosher salt& black pepper

Instructions

1. Soak wooden skewers in up to 30 minutes before using. Heat the grill to medium-high.
2. Place the zucchini, onions, mushrooms, and lemon pieces on each skewer.
3. Whisk together the oil, herbs, garlic, and red pepper flakes in a small bowl. Season skewers with pepper and salt after brushing them all over.
4. Cook for 12 to 14 minutes, occasionally rotating, until veggies are soft and slightly charred. Serve immediately.

Grilled Cabbage Steaks

(Ready in about 30 minutes | serving 4|Difficulty: Easy)

Per serving: Kcal 66.9, Fat: 2.1g, Net Carbs: 11.6g, Protein: 3.1g

Ingredients

- 1 large cabbage head, cut into ½ inch pieces
- Olive oil (extra-virgin) for brushing
- Kosher salt & black pepper
- Red pepper flakes 1 pinch, crushed
- Cooked bacon, chopped for serving
- Blue cheese, crumbled for serving
- Green onions, freshly chopped for serving
- For serving, ranch dressing

Instructions

1. Preheat the grill to medium-high. Season with pepper, salt, and red pepper flakes on both sides of the cabbage steaks. Cook until soft, about five minutes per side, on the grill.
2. Before serving, top with blue cheese, bacon, and scallions, then drizzle with ranch dressing.

Zucchini and Cauliflower Skewers with Feta

(Ready in about 20 minutes | serving 6|Difficulty: Easy)

Per serving: Kcal 119, Fat: 8g, Net Carbs: 12g, Protein: 3g

Ingredients

- Zucchini & summer squash, 4 large
- Cauliflower 1 head, cut into florets
- Skewers 8, soaked in water for twenty minutes
- Olive oil (extra-virgin) for drizzling
- Kosher salt & black pepper
- Crumbled feta 1/4 cup

Instructions

1. Preheat the grill to medium-high temperature. Using a Y peeler or a mandolin, shave yellow squash and zucchini into long strips. Yellow squash, Zucchini, and cauliflower should all be skewered. Season with pepper and salt and drizzle with olive oil.
2. Grill, rotating periodically, for 10 to 12 minutes, or until veggies are soft and slightly charred.
3. Toss with feta cheese.

Charred Green Beans with Ricotta and Lemon

(Ready in about 15 minutes | serving 4|Difficulty: Easy)

Per serving: Kcal 208, Fat: 14g, Net Carbs: 12.9g, Protein: 9g

Ingredients

- Green beans 1 1/2 lbs., trimmed
- Ricotta (whole-milk) 2 cups
- 3 tbsp. Olive oil (extra-virgin), plus more for drizzling
- Kosher salt 3/4 tsp, plus more
- 1 tsp lemon zest, finely grated
- Black pepper, freshly ground
- For serving, lemon wedges

Instructions

1. Preheat the grill to medium-high. Place green beans on a hot grill if using a grill. Cover and grill for about 8 minutes, rotating once halfway through, till beans are slightly charred and crisp-tender.
2. Meanwhile, in a large mixing bowl, whisk 3 tbsp. oil, ricotta, and 3/4 tsp. salt with an electric mixer at medium-high speed until thick and creamy, about 2 minutes.
3. Arrange charred green beans on top of whipped ricotta on a serving plate. Season with pepper and salt after drizzling with oil and lemon zest. Serve with lemon slices on the side.

Grilled Beet Salad with Burrata and Cherries

(Ready in about 1 hour 20 minutes | serving 4|Difficulty: Easy)

Per serving: Kcal 273, Fat: 21g, Net Carbs: 17.5g, Protein: 5.6g

Ingredients

- 2 lb. Each beet 6 medium
- Sherry vinegar 1 tbsp.
- Kosher salt 1 tsp.
- 3 tbsp. Olive oil (extra-virgin), plus more for drizzling
- Mozzarella 8 oz., slice into 2-inch pieces
- Fresh cherries 8 oz., halved & pitted
- Castelvetrano olives 1 cup, smashed & pitted
- Salt & black pepper, freshly ground

Instructions

1. In a grill, prepare a charcoal fire. Allow the coals to cool to medium heat.
2. Grill beets directly over coals, occasionally rotating, for 35–45 minutes, or until skins are charred and flesh is fork-tender. (Alternatively, cook 45–55 minutes on the grate of a gas/charcoal grill, covered, over medium-high heat, rotating regularly.) Cover tightly using plastic wrap and place in a large mixing bowl. Allow to steam until it is safe to handle.
3. Pull charred skins from beets (they should fall off easily), and slice each beet into Six wedges while wearing gloves if you don't want pink hands. Toss with kosher salt, vinegar, and 3 tablespoons oil in a large mixing dish.
4. Arrange the beets on a serving plate. Cherries, Burrata, and olives go on top. Season with sea pepper and salt after drizzling with oil.

Charred Leeks with Honey and Vinegar

(Ready in about 35 minutes | serving 4|Difficulty: Easy)

Per serving: Kcal 112, Fat: 8g, Net Carbs: 12g, Protein: 4g

Ingredients

- 2 ½ lb. Each leek 4 medium, white & pale green parts only
- Red wine vinegar 2 tbsp.
- Honey 2 tsp.
- 2 tbsp. Olive oil (extra-virgin), plus more for drizzling
- Kosher salt & freshly ground pepper

Instructions

1. Heat a grill to a high temperature. Remove any sand or dirt from the leeks and pat them dry. Grill, rotating every few minutes with tongs until outsides are thoroughly charred for 12–16 minutes.
2. Place the leeks on a cutting board and set them aside for 10 minutes.
3. While leeks are resting, combine the honey and vinegar in a small bowl and whisk until the honey is completely dissolved. Set aside the dressing.
4. On a diagonal, cut the leeks into 112"–2" pieces. Mix with 2 tbsp. oil in a medium mixing bowl and season with salt.
5. Place the leeks on a plate and drizzle with the remaining dressing. Season with salt and pepper and drizzle with additional oil.

Grilled Watermelon, Feta, and Tomato Salad

(Ready in about 25 minutes | serving 4|Difficulty: Easy)

Per serving: Kcal 314, Fat: 8.5g, Net Carbs: 60.7g, Protein: 6.9g

Ingredients

- Olive oil 1 tbsp., plus more
- 1 seedless watermelon (4-pound), rind removed & sliced
- Kosher salt 1 tsp, divided
- Heirloom tomatoes 4 multicolored, thinly sliced
- 1/2 tsp black pepper, freshly ground plus more
- 1 ¼ cup Feta 6 ounces, thinly sliced

Instructions

1. Preheat a grill to medium-high and oil the grate.
2. Cut watermelon into circles with a 2" diameter ring cutter or a thin drinking glass; you must have 20–22 slices. Sprinkle 1/2 tsp salt on both sides of the watermelon. Watermelon should be grilled until nicely charred on both sides, about two minutes per side. Transfer to a dish and set aside for 10 minutes, or till cool to the touch.
3. In a large mixing bowl, combine tomatoes, 1 tsp salt, 1 tbsp. oil, and 1/2 tsp pepper.
4. On a dish, alternate layers of the tomato mixture, watermelon, and cheese draining any excess liquid from tomatoes before using. Serve with a drizzle of oil and a pinch of black pepper.

Grilled Corn with Hot Paprika Oil and Manchego Cheese

(Ready in about 25 minutes | serving 4|Difficulty: Easy)

Per serving: Kcal 116, Fat: 4g, Net Carbs: 12g, Protein: 2g

Ingredients

- Lime 1
- 3 corn ears, husks & silk removed
- Hot pimentón, 1 tsp (smoked paprika)
- 4 tsp olive oil (extra-virgin)
- Aged manchego cheese 1 ounce
- Sea salt

Instructions

1. Preheat the grill to high heat.
2. Remove the lime's top and bottom. Remove the zest and set it aside. To get the lime segments out of the membranes, cut between them. Place in a large mixing bowl and set aside. Grill the corn for about 5 minutes, occasionally rotating to ensure even charring. Cut the kernels off cobs when they are cool enough to handle. Toss with the lime segments in the mixing bowl until fully mixed. Serve in separate serving bowls.
3. In a small dish, combine the oil and pimentón and drizzle over the corn. With a Microplane, shave some cheese directly over the corn mixture, then add the lime zest on top. Serve immediately with a pinch of Maldon salt.

Red Curry–Marinated Japanese Eggplant

(Ready in about 35 minutes | serving 4|Difficulty: Easy)

Per serving: Kcal 57, Fat: 3.4g, Net Carbs: 6.4g, Protein: 1.6g

Ingredients

- Fresno chiles 6, seeds removed
- Garlic 4 cloves
- Lemongrass stalks 2, finely grated
- Vegetable oil 1/3 cup
- 1 tbsp. Peeled ginger, finely grated
- 1 tsp cumin, ground
- Sugar 1/2 tsp
- Kosher salt 1 tsp, plus more
- Japanese eggplants 4, halved lengthwise

Instructions

1. In a food processor, puree the chiles, lemongrass, garlic, oil, cumin, ginger, sugar, and 1 tsp salt until smooth. With the blade of a sharp knife, score the sliced sides of the eggplant in the cross-hatch pattern. Add a generous amount of curry paste to each eggplant and set aside any leftover paste. Allow at least ten minutes or up to 1 hour for the eggplants to sit.

2. Preheat the grill to medium-high. Season eggplants lightly with salt and grill for 5 minutes per side, frequently flipping, until browned and soft. Serve with the curry paste that has been set aside.

PART 6: SAUCES, MARINADES & RUBS

Rosemary Garlic Rub

(Ready in about 5 minutes | serving 4|Difficulty: Easy)

Per serving: Kcal 177, Fat: 18.3g, Net Carbs: 3.8g, Protein: 0.6g

Ingredients

- Black pepper 1 tbsp. Ground
- 1 tbsp. Kosher salt
- 3 tbsp. Rosemary, chopped & fresh
- 1 tbsp. Dried rosemary
- Garlic 8 cloves, diced
- Olive oil ⅓ cup

Instructions

1. Combine black pepper, fresh rosemary, kosher salt, dried rosemary, and garlic in a small bowl. Stir with just enough olive oil to make a thick paste. Before grilling, rub desired meats.

Advice:

This olive oil-based rub is fantastic on pork or chicken, especially when grilled indirectly. This works well with potatoes as well.

Jerk seasoning

(Ready in about 10 minutes | serving 1|Difficulty: Easy)

Per serving: Kcal 304, Fat: 28.4g, Net Carbs: 15g, Protein: 1.8g

Ingredients

- 2 tbsp. Onion, dried & minced
- 2 ½ tsp thyme, dried
- 2 tsp ground allspice
- 2 tsp black pepper, ground
- ½ tsp cinnamon, ground
- Cayenne pepper ½ tsp
- Salt ½ tsp
- Vegetable oil 2 tbsp.

Instructions

1. Combine the dried onion, allspice, thyme, ground black pepper, cayenne pepper, cinnamon, and salt in a small bowl. Rub spice onto meat after lightly coating it in oil.

Advice:

This seasoning is fantastic on any meat. You can make a larger batch and keep it in an airtight container.

Carolina-Style Barbeque Sauce

(Ready in about 45 minutes | serving 4|Difficulty: Easy)

Per serving: Kcal 52, Fat: 0.9g, Net Carbs: 9.8g, Protein: 0.6g

Ingredients

- Vegetable oil ½ tsp
- Peeled apple 1, cored & chopped
- Brown sugar 2 tbsp.
- Apple cider vinegar 1 cup
- Yellow mustard 2 tbsp.
- Red pepper flakes 1 tbsp., or to taste
- Black pepper 1 tbsp. Ground

Instructions

1. In a medium saucepan, heat the oil. Cook and stir the apple pieces in a saucepan until they have been slightly caramelized for about two minutes.
2. Cook, constantly stirring, till the mixture begins to boil, about 2 minutes.
3. Fill a saucepan halfway with apple cider vinegar. Reduce to a low heat setting and cover. Cook for 30 minutes, or until apples are tender and falling apart. Remove the pan from the heat.
4. Combine the red pepper flakes, mustard, and black pepper in a mixing bowl.
5. Puree the contents in a blender until it is perfectly smooth.

Advice:

Fresh apple is featured in this Carolina-style barbecue sauce, but it's a simple tart dish. It's delicious on pulled pork & pork chops marinated in molasses.

Italian Chicken Marinade

(Ready in about 4 hours 30 minutes | serving 4|Difficulty: Difficult)

Per serving: Kcal 455, Fat: 34.2g, Net Carbs: 12g, Protein: 25.1g

Ingredients

- 1 bottle salad dressing, Italian-style (16 ounces)
- 1 tsp garlic powder
- 1 tsp salt
- 4 halved chicken breast, skinless & boneless

Instructions

1. Combine the garlic powder, salad dressing, and salt in a deep baking dish. Place the chicken in the bowl and toss it around to evenly coat it. Refrigerate for at least four hours before serving. (For optimal results, marinate for at least 24 hours.)
2. Preheat the grill to medium-high.
3. Grates should be lightly oiled. Remove the chicken from the marinade and cook for 6-8 minutes on each side, or till juices run clear.

Advice:

This is a fast and easy way to marinate your chicken.

Best Pork Chop Marinade

(Ready in about 6 hours 10 minutes | serving 2|Difficulty: Difficult)

Per serving: Kcal 756, Fat: 41.6g, Net Carbs: 29.6g, Protein: 62.1g

Ingredients

- Pork chops 2 large
- ¼ cup olive oil (extra-virgin)
- 3 tbsp. Dark brown sugar
- 2 tbsp. Lemon juice
- Spicy brown mustard 2 tbsp.
- Garlic 4 cloves, chopped
- Dried thyme 2 tsp
- Onion powder 1 tsp
- Worcestershire sauce 1 tsp
- White wine vinegar 1 tsp
- Mesquite flavored seasoning 1 tsp
- Parsley flakes ½ tsp dried
- ½ tsp kosher salt
- ½ tsp black pepper, freshly ground

Instructions

1. Each pork chop should be cut horizontally from one side to the center within 2 inches of the other side. Open the two sides like a book and spread them out.

2. In a big resealable plastic bag, combine olive oil, lemon juice, brown sugar, mustard, garlic, onion powder, thyme, Worcestershire sauce, mesquite seasoning, vinegar, parsley, pepper, and salt. Add the pork chops to the bag, coat them in the marinade, push out any excess air, and seal it. Refrigerate for 6 - 8 hours to marinate.

Advice: It is best for pork chops.

Homemade Kansas City-Style BBQ Sauce

(Ready in about 1 hour 10 minutes | serving 4|Difficulty: Easy)

Per serving: Kcal 152, Fat: 0g, Net Carbs: 39g, Protein: 0g

Ingredients

- Ketchup 1 1/2 cup
- Brown sugar 1 cup, packed
- Water 1/2 cup
- Apple cider vinegar 1/4 cup
- Worcestershire sauce 1 tbsp.
- Molasses 1 tbsp.
- Kosher salt 1 tsp.
- Garlic powder 1/2 tsp.
- Onion powder 1/2 tsp.
- Ground mustard 1/4 tsp.
- Paprika 1/4 tsp.

Instructions

1. Whisk all of the ingredients together in a small saucepan over medium heat.

Bring the mixture to a boil, gradually reduce to low heat and cook, stirring periodically, for 45 minutes, or until thickened.

Allow cooling at room temperature before storing in an airtight jar in the refrigerator.

Advice:

This barbecue sauce is fantastic on almost anything. Pizza, grilled chicken, and even nachos are favorites.

Homemade Taco Seasoning

(Ready in about 5 minutes | serving 4|Difficulty: Easy)

Per serving: Kcal 8.9, Fat: 0.2g, Net Carbs: 2g, Protein: 0.4g

Ingredients

Chili powder 2 tbsp.

Ground cumin 1 tbsp.

Smoked paprika 1 1/2 tsp.

Garlic powder 1 tsp.

Onion powder 1 tsp.

Salt 1 tsp.

Black pepper 1 tsp.

Dried oregano 1/2 tsp.

Instructions

Combine all ingredients in a small bowl. Place in an airtight jar to keep fresh.

Advice:

This homemade taco seasoning recipe is simple to make and goes well for everything from tacos to vegetables, soups, meat, rice, seafood, beans, soups, salads, and more.

Chili Garlic Chicken Wings Rub

(Ready in about 3 hours 20 minutes| serving 4|Difficulty: Moderate)

Per serving: Kcal 132.5, Fat: 5.9g, Net Carbs: 5g, Protein: 15.4g

Ingredients

1/3 cup olive oil (extra-virgin)

1/3 cup soy sauce (low-sodium)

Honey 1/4 cup

Chili garlic sauce 1/4 cup

1 lime juice

Garlic 4 cloves, minced

1 tbsp. Ginger, freshly minced

Chicken wings 2 lb.

Instructions

Whisk together the oil, honey, soy sauce, chili garlic sauce, garlic, lime juice, and ginger in a large mixing bowl. Rub it on chicken before grilling.

Advice:

It goes well with cheesy taco casserole, taco tomatoes, and cheesy chicken pasta. To be honest, this would probably enhance the flavor of any vegetable or meat.

Chicago Steakhouse Rub

(Ready in about 5 minutes| serving 4|Difficulty: Easy)

Per serving: Kcal 0, Fat: 0g, Net Carbs: 0g, Protein: 0g

Ingredients

Granulated garlic 1 tbsp.

Kosher salt 2 tbsp.

Black pepper 1 tbsp. Coarsely ground

Flank steak 1 1 1/2 lbs., at room temperature

Evoo

Instructions

Combine salt, garlic, and pepper in a mixing bowl. Before grilling, brush meat with EVOO, brush with rub, and pat to adhere.

Advice:

It is great on pork roasts, ribs, and vegetables.

Guinness Marinade

(Ready in about 5 minutes| serving 4|Difficulty: Easy)

Per serving: Kcal 50, Fat: 0g, Net Carbs: 13g, Protein: 0g

Ingredients

Guinness 14.9 ounces

EVOO 1/3 cup, plus more for brushing

Onion 1 red, cut into rounds

2 tbsp. Flat-leaf parsley, chopped

1 flank steak 1 1/2 lbs., at room temperature

Instructions

Combine 1/3 cup EVOO, Guinness, onion, and parsley in a mixing bowl. Add the steak and marinate for 30 minutes in the refrigerator. Before grilling, pat dry, brush with EVOO, and season with salt & pepper. If desired, grill onions with the steak.

Advice:

It is best for chicken, meat steaks, salmon and oysters.

PART 7: SIDE DISHES

Grilled Potato Fans with Onions

(Ready in about 55 minutes| serving 4|Difficulty: Easy)

Per serving: Kcal 302, Fat: 13g, Net Carbs: 41g, Protein: 7g

Ingredients

Potatoes 6 medium

Onions 2 small, halved & thinly sliced

Butter 6 tbsp., diced

Garlic 2 cloves, minced

Parmesan cheese 6 tbsp., grated

1 tbsp. Chives, minced

1/2 tsp red pepper flakes, crushed

Dash salt

Instructions

Make sure the grill is set to indirect heat. Cut each potato into 1/2-inch slices with a sharp knife, leaving the pieces attached at the bottom. Potatoes should be lightly brushed. Each one should be placed on a 12-inch piece of heavy-duty foil.

Between the potatoes slices, place the butter, onions, and garlic. Sprinkle the cheese, pepper flakes, chives, and salt between the slices. Fold the foil around the potatoes and seal it tightly.

Cover and cook for 35-45 minutes over indirect medium heat or until tender. Carefully open the foil to let steam escape.

Grilled Pattypans

(Ready in about 15 minutes| serving 4|Difficulty: Easy)

Per serving: Kcal 54, Fat: 0g, Net Carbs: 12g, Protein: 1g

Ingredients

1 ½ lb. Pattypan squash 6 cups

Apricot fruit 1/4 cup

Hoisin sauce 2 tsp

Rice vinegar 1 tsp

Sesame oil ½ tsp

Salt ¼ tsp

Ground ginger 1/8 tsp

Instructions

Place the squash in a grill wok that has been sprayed with cooking spray. Grill for 4 minutes on each side, covered, over medium-high heat till tender.

Meanwhile, add the remaining ingredients to a small bowl. Transfer the squash to a serving dish and stir gently with the sauce.

Herbed Butternut Squash

(Ready in about 20 minutes| serving 4|Difficulty: Easy)

Per serving: Kcal 108, Fat: 2g, Net Carbs: 23g, Protein: 2g

Ingredients

3 lbs. Butternut squash 1 medium

Olive oil 1 tbsp.

Dried oregano 1 ½ tsp

Dried thyme 1 tsp

Salt 1/2 tsp

Pepper 1/4 tsp

Instructions

Squash should be peeled and cut crosswise into 1/2-inch thick slices; seeds should be removed and discarded. Toss the squash with the remaining ingredients in a large mixing bowl. Grill 7-8 minutes on each side, covered, over medium-high heat 4 inches from heat until tender.

Fingerling Potatoes with Fresh Parsley and Chives

(Ready in about 40 minutes| serving 4|Difficulty: Easy)

Per serving: Kcal 215, Fat: 9g, Net Carbs: 30g, Protein: 4g

Ingredients

Fingerling potatoes 2 lbs.

Olive oil 1/4 cup

Goya sazon (without annatto) 1/2 tsp

Adobo seasoning 1/2 tsp

2 tbsp. Parsley, minced & fresh

2 tbsp. Chives, minced

Instructions

In a 6-quart stockpot, place the potatoes and enough water to cover them. Bring the water to a boil. Reduce heat to low and simmer, uncovered, for 16-20 minutes or till vegetables are soft. Drain the water. Combine olive oil & seasonings in a large mixing bowl; set aside 1 tablespoon. Toss in the potatoes to coat. Allow 15 minutes for cooling.

Four metal or moistened wooden skewers, threaded with potatoes. Cook for 8-10 minutes, covered, over medium-high heat until browned, flipping once. Allow cooling slightly.

Remove the skewers from the potatoes. Place the potatoes in a large mixing bowl. Toss in the herbs and the leftover marinade.

Quick Barbecued Beans

(Ready in about 25 minutes| serving 4|Difficulty: Easy)

Per serving: Kcal 264, Fat: 2g, Net Carbs: 51g, Protein: 14g

Ingredients

1 can kidney beans (16 ounces), rinsed & drained

1 can great northern beans (15 ½ ounces), rinsed & drained

1 can pork & beans (15 ounces)

Barbecue sauce 1/2 cup

Brown sugar 2 tbsp.

Prepared mustard 2 tsp

Instructions

Combine all ingredients in an oiled grill pan.

Cook, covered, over medium-high heat for 15-20 minutes, or until well cooked, stirring occasionally.

Blue Cheese & Bacon Stuffed Peppers

(Ready in about 20 minutes| serving 4|Difficulty: Easy)

Per serving: Kcal 73, Fat: 6g, Net Carbs: 3g, Protein: 3g

Ingredients

Sweet orange, yellow, or red peppers 3 medium

Cream cheese 4 ounces, softened

Crumbled blue cheese 1/2 cup

Bacon 3 strips, cooked & crumbled

Onion 1 green, thinly sliced

Instructions

Peppers should be quartered. Stems and seeds should be removed and discarded. Mix blue cheese, cream cheese, bacon, and green onion in a

small mixing bowl.

Cover and grill peppers over medium heat 4 inches away from heat until lightly charred, 3-4 minutes per side.

Remove the peppers from the grill and stuff them with about 1 spoonful of the cheese mixture each. Grill for another 2-3 minutes, or until the cheese has melted.

Grilled Corn Medley

(Ready in about 20 minutes| serving 4|Difficulty: Easy)

Per serving: Kcal 83, Fat: 4.6g, Net Carbs: 9.2g, Protein: 2.2g

Ingredients

Corn ears 3 medium, sweet cut into 2-inch bits

Red pepper 1 medium, sweet cut into 1-inch bits

Zucchini, 1 medium sliced

Fresh mushrooms 20 small

Caesar salad dressing 1/4 cup, creamy

Salt 1/4 tsp

Pepper 1/4 tsp

Instructions

Combine all ingredients in a large mixing bowl and toss to coat. Transfer to a foil pan that can be discarded. Cover and cook for 5 minutes over medium-high heat, stirring occasionally. Grill for another 3-5 minutes, or until the vegetables are tender.

Rice on the Grill

(Ready in about 30 minutes| serving 4|Difficulty: Easy)

Per serving: Kcal 104, Fat: 2g, Net Carbs: 21g, Protein: 2g

Ingredients

1 1/3 cups instant rice, uncooked

1/3 cup mushrooms, sliced & fresh

1/4 cup green pepper, chopped

1/4 cup onion, chopped

Water 1/2 cup

Chicken broth 1/2 cup

Ketchup 1/3 cup

Butter 1 tbsp.

Instructions

Mix the first seven ingredients in a 9-inch round disposable foil pan. Make a butter spread. Place on a grill on medium-high heat.

Cover and cook for 12-15 minutes over medium heat or till liquid is absorbed. Carefully remove the foil to enable steam to escape. Using a fork, fluff the mix.

Corn 'n' Squash Quesadillas

(Ready in about 50 minutes| serving 4|Difficulty: Easy)

Per serving: Kcal 301, Fat: 12g, Net Carbs: 38g, Protein: 11g

Ingredients

Sweet corn ears 2 medium, husks removed

Halved summer squash 2 medium, yellow

Sweet onion 1/2 small, cut into ¼ inch pieces

Jalapeno peppers 2

Basil, 1 tbsp. Minced & fresh

Oregano 1-1/2 tsp, minced & fresh

Garlic 1 clove, minced

Salt 1/4 tsp

Ground cumin 1/4 tsp

8-inch flour tortillas 6, warmed

Monterey jack cheese 1 cup, shredded

Canola oil 1 tbsp.

Instructions

Cover and grill corn for 10 minutes over medium heat; turn. Cover and cook the onion, squash, and jalapenos for 4-6 minutes on each side on the grill. Remove the corn from cobs, cut the squash & onion, and seed and cut the jalapenos after the vegetables are cool to the touch. Place in a big mixing bowl. Combine the basil, garlic, oregano, salt, and cumin in a mixing bowl. On one side of each tortilla, spread 1/2 cup filling; top with cheese. Tortillas should be folded over the filling. Cook quesadillas in oil in a large cast-iron skillet or griddle over medium-high heat until heated through, about 1-2 minutes per side. Cut the wedges in half.

Pimento Pasta Salad

(Ready in about 15 minutes| serving 4|Difficulty: Easy)

Per serving: Kcal 313, Fat: 17g, Net Carbs: 29g, Protein: 10g

Ingredients

Elbow macaroni 1 lb.

Pimento peppers 3 jars, drained

Shredded cheddar 2 cup

Mayonnaise 3/4 cup

Cayenne pepper 1 tsp.

Kosher salt

Chopped chives 1/4 cup

Instructions

Cook macaroni until al dente in a large pot with salted boiling water according to package guidelines. Drain the water and set it aside.

Combine macaroni, cheddar, peppers, mayonnaise, and cayenne pepper in a large mixing bowl. Mix thoroughly. To taste, season with salt.

Serve with chives as a garnish.

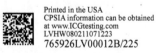

Printed in the USA
CPSIA information can be obtained
at www.ICGtesting.com
LVHW080211071223
765926LV00012B/225

9 781803 431765